The Five Health Frontiers

'A brilliant exposé of how the political left in Britain is unaware of, and can start to begin to address, the effects of ever-increasing opting-out from public health and care services by those who can.'

—Danny Dorling, Professor of Geography, University of Oxford

'The boldest blueprint for public health since Bevan.'

—Sonia Adesara, NHS Doctor and Campaigner

'The ideas in this book are as significant and radical as the birth of the NHS, it shows a new, fairer vision for improving the health of the nation and a comprehensive plan for how to do it.'

—Shirley Cramer, former CEO of the Royal Society for Public Health

'A vital book that shows just how broken the health status quo truly is. Thomas's work will arm campaigners to demand a better, more just public health system – and to defend human life against corporate exploitation.'

—Dr Aseem Malhotra, author of *A Statin-Free Life* and Founder of Public Health Collaboration

'A well-argued plan to bring together health, social and economic justice.'

—Andy McDonald MP

The Five Health Frontiers

A New Radical Blueprint

Christopher Thomas

PLUTO PRESS

First published 2022 by Pluto Press
New Wing, Somerset House, Strand, London WC2R 1LA

www.plutobooks.com

British Library Cataloguing in Publication Data
A catalogue record for this book is available from the British Library

ISBN   978 0 7453 4393 8   Hardback
ISBN   978 0 7453 4392 1   Paperback
ISBN   978 0 7453 4395 2   PDF
ISBN   978 0 7453 4394 5   EPUB

This book is printed on paper suitable for recycling and made from fully managed and sustained forest sources. Logging, pulping and manufacturing processes are expected to conform to the environmental standards of the country of origin.

Typeset by Stanford DTP Services, Northampton, England

Simultaneously printed in the United Kingdom and United States of America

Contents

'Salus Populi Suprema Lex Esto'
The health of the people should be the supreme law
Marcus Tullius Cicero

To Alex

Abbreviations

A&E	Accident and Emergency
ADASS	Association of Directors of Adult Social Services
CSR	Corporate Social Responsibility
CQC	Care Quality Commission
DHSC	Department of Health and Social Care
DWP	Department for Work and Pensions
GHSI	Global Health Security Index
GND	Green New Deal
GNP	Gross National Product
IEA	Institute of Economic Affairs
IPPR	Institute for Public Policy Research
MHCLG	Ministry of Housing, Communities and Local Government
NCS	National Care Service
NEF	New Economics Foundation
NHS	National Health Service
NICE	The National Institute for Health and Care Excellence
NILSS	National Independent Living Support Service
NPM	New Public Management
OECD	The Organisation for Economic Co-operation and Development
OFG	Office for Future Generations
ONS	Office for National Statistics
PFI	Private Finance Initiative(s)
PHE	Public Health England
PHND	Public Health New Deal
PHN-ZERO	Public Health Net Zero
SAGE	Scientific Advisory Group on Emergencies
SDIL	Soft Drinks Industry Levy
TB	Tuberculosis
TUC	Trade Unions Congress
UTB	Universalise the Best

List of Tables

Acknowledgements

It's not always easy to write a book about health during a health crisis. Combining a day job researching health and care with evenings and weekends spent thinking and writing about the implications of the pandemic could at times be oppressive. There were moments I wanted nothing more than to stop, hide away and think about anything else. But this has been a universal experience for many of us over the last 15 months, each witness to the deadly nature of the pandemic and the personal cost of failures in government policy.

In other moments, I felt incredibly privileged. Privileged to have had the opportunity to channel my fear and frustration into the catharsis of imagining what radical change must now follow – and might just become possible. There are few better coping mechanisms.

I could not be more grateful to Pluto Press for publishing this book. Neda Tehrani was an immediate champion for my book from the proposal. She has pushed it in ambition, scope and relevance ever since, for which I'm hugely grateful. Others have made huge contributions throughout the writing process. I appreciate the feedback given by my parents, by Harry Quilter-Pinner at the IPPR on an early draft, and from many others who read chapters or who listened to me read it out loud.

This book would not have been possible without the immense work from the academic and policy community. I am lucky to be able to draw from such a large base of fascinating research and scholarship – it's a book built on the shoulders of giants. I hope what follows does some justice in translating our fantastic evidence into big policy ideas.

Most of all, though, my thanks to Alex – who has managed to be my partner while I dedicated weekends, evenings and early mornings to writing this book over the last 18 months. There is an irony that the health consequences of stress, overwork and burnout are covered in some detail – but she helped ensure I got through all these experiences safe and sound. Sometimes there has been joy, and sometimes it has been a dark and frustrating process. For being there and sharing in both, thank you.

Preface

The idea for this book came well before Covid-19. For a few years, I'd had a half-written book proposal saved in an out-the-way part of my computer. It emerged from my growing sense that there was something deeply wrong with how our public health system works – a fundamental discordance between health today and the democratic socialist ideals upon which the National Health Service (NHS) was founded in 1948.

Often, we chalk 'health' up in the left-wing win column. We talk lovingly about the UK's system of universal care, based on need rather than identity, income, or ability to pay. But the brutal reality is that our public health system still distributes the best health to the people with the most money or power, and the worst health to the poorest and most marginalised.

Today, the most disadvantaged people in our country struggle most to access the healthcare that they need, and experience substantially worse outcomes when it comes to both length and quality of life. These injustices were not eradicated by the advent of the NHS – and they have been observed both in periods in which the health service has had plenty, and in periods where it has been starved of funding.

When news first broke of a new infectious disease spreading across the world, in the first days of 2020, I remember feeling confident we'd be okay. The UK was in an incredibly privileged position. We're an advanced economy, we're an island, we had a well-regarded infectious disease surveillance system, we have universal healthcare, people aren't denied tests, vaccines, or treatments as a rule, and we have an influential role in the global health system.[1]

It quickly became clear that any such confidence was misplaced. To the horror of most in the health, medical and scientific communities – as well as the public – almost everything that could go wrong, did go wrong. Communication was poor and action was often lagging. In March 2020, large sporting and music events carried on, even as infection rates climbed. Lockdowns were repeatedly implemented too late. 'Test and Trace' was established, cancelled, re-announced and then outsourced to disastrous consequence and cost. All the while, tens of thousands of people died.

In an article on *The Plague*, Jacqueline Rose describes Albert Camus' presentation of 'the pestilence' as both 'blight and revelation'.[2] My revelation from this pestilence was that, while exasperated by bad policy decisions during the pandemic itself, many of the problems we faced weren't new. Rather, Covid-19 exposed and exploited structural problems that already existed, only now at a huge scale. In many cases, those structural problems were the same as the ones I had written of in my half-written book proposal.

In some parts, this book tells a story of the discrepancy between the NHS as it exists today, and the intentions and principles set out by Nye Bevan when he founded the service in the late 1940s. But it is quite a different story to the one told in the health books that have come before it. Often, interventions that cover the health service only take aim at the failures of neoliberals, libertarians, conservatives and right-wingers – usually, by sounding the alarm about privatisation. By contrast, this book is just as interested in taking a critical look at the left's strategies to 'save' our NHS. Specifically, it asks why the stories we tell – and the perennial rear-guard action we employ to defend against the wrecking ball of privatisation – are no longer proving either effective or sustainable.

And while it would be difficult to write a book on health without talking about the NHS, I am of the strong opinion that this book is most important when it doesn't talk about the health service at all. Our love of the NHS – 'the closest thing the English people have to a religion', to quote Nigel Lawson – has led to what I call an 'NHS-centrism' on the left. 'NHS' and health have become nearly synonymous among the public, politicians, journalists and activists. But if our goal is to advance health improvement and address health justice, this is far from optimal.

Though it's not a recent finding, it still surprises people I talk to just how much of our health is defined outside of brick-and-mortar hospitals and Accident and Emergency (A&E) departments. Just 10 to 20 per cent of the disparities between people's health outcomes are explained by differential access to healthcare. The other 80 to 90 per cent are explained by factors like our environment, our socio-economic status, or the places that we live in – that is, by our material conditions. This brings into scope agendas and policy levers far beyond the NHS or the Department of Health and Social Care.

To really get to grips with the big questions in health – why life expectancy is stalling, why health inequality is widening, why pandemics are breaking out, why the global health system is increasingly vulnerable and why policy doesn't seem to be making a blind bit of difference – the left needs to expand the passion we have for our universal health service to the other key pillars of the public health system. We need to look at how we've failed to inoculate people against the health consequences of social injustice, and the way poverty expresses itself on our bodies as ill health. We need to look at how we have allowed businesses to profit at the expense of our health, without penalty or shame. We need to look at how a nationalistic approach to health placed us at risk of major health shocks and how it continues to do so. Each of these points is covered by a chapter in this book.

In some cases, the book adds value by highlighting new evidence on key aspects of health improvement or health justice. But, while I have aimed to give attention to drivers of poor and unequal health that traditionally receive less attention, I realise that the evidence on the drivers of poor health is very well established elsewhere, too. This book owes a clear debt to the writers on health inequalities that have come before: Kate Pickett, Richard Wilkinson, Michael Marmot, Lee Humber, David Stuckler, Sanjay Basu, Danny Dorling and others. There are perhaps, then, two places where this book adds value in places less well covered by other works. First, it applies a distinctly radical framing. A key objective here is to bring public health within the scope of the left's wider search for a cogent, coherent and compelling political project that is built around justice.[3] Too often, I find, the health sector and the progressive sector have very separate conversations, using disparate languages – and this book helps to bridge the gap between the two in a post-pandemic moment when our ambitions are broadly aligned.

Second, this book recognises that for all our evidence there is a poverty of radical, left-wing policy thinking in health. The sad truth is that there hasn't really been an exciting health policy since the 1948 National Health Service Act and – for pockets of promising work – health has not hosted the same levels of creativity and ambition as agendas like economic, climate and criminal justice. Now more than ever, we desperately need exciting ideas that explain why public health is important, and why it can be a keystone in a compelling vision of a better future.

In line with that ambition, this book adopts the broadest possible definition of 'public health'. For some, public health means a limited array of local and community services, funded out by a small ring-fenced grant. But in this book, it refers to everything that contributes both to the aggregate health of the population and the way that stock of health is shared out. Public health in this book is therefore not a single arm of the welfare state, but rather a comprehensive and distributive system (akin to the economy). Defined in this way, public health can provide an anchor for a holistic vision for our society and economy – perhaps even an alternative to GDP more suited to the left's goals and agenda.

In thinking about how the left achieve change, I often refer to progressive, left or otherwise grassroot social movements. A key reason for writing this book is to undertake a constructive exploration of the state of the thinking, politics and campaigning around health on the left. Given that, I want to be clear from the outset: I realise the progressive movement is creative, diverse and often in productive disagreement with itself. I therefore realise that when I talk about the 'mainstream', it might lead me to overstate the homogeneity – and that for any critique I put forward, there will be grassroot exceptions. I've aimed to counterbalance this by pointing out a selection of the great examples of activism that do exist in the grassroots. But my main interest is with the mainstream: which left health arguments and topics receive the most bandwidth, the most attention, the most voluntary time and the most funding. Far from erasing the places that are good, my hope is this contribution strengthens the best of the vital work going on in the grassroots.

Another phrase I use regularly throughout the book is 'health justice' – a lesser heard term within the health sector today. More often, we use the language of 'health inequality', 'inequity', or 'the social determinants of health'. We could get lost in semantics here, and I have seen whole programmes of what could have been worthwhile work derailed by an inability to pick a term. I've chosen health justice as it feels better aligned to one of my core propositions: that when it comes to health, we need to be more interested in how power operates, and more cognisant of how we align to other movements focused on radical change and societal justice.

The overwhelming message is one of optimism. I believe that through collaboration, the destruction wreaked by Covid can be the ashes from which the phoenix of better health rises. While we cannot dodge the brutal reality of fundamental problems with the health status quo, this book seeks to provide a new, radical blueprint – one through which public health and care can provide the foundation for a fairer society for all.

Introduction

In February 1928, George Orwell – or Eric Blair as he was then still known – arrived in Paris. He was not alone in yielding to the allures of the city of lights. It was then home to a number of his literary contemporaries – Gertrude Stein, T.S. Eliot, Jean Rhys, Ernest Hemingway and Ezra Pound all among them.

For many, the draw of Paris was the hedonistic 'café culture' of the inter-war period – an appropriate environment for the cultivation of literary bohemianism and high-minded modernist prose. This was not to be Orwell's experience. Instead, his stay in the city would be defined by the shock of a sudden and severe illness.

This experience of ill health would stay with Orwell throughout his life. In the immediate aftermath, the experience informed the semi-fictional *Down and Out in Paris and London* (1933).[1] Twenty years later, he returned to the period, this time in the non-fiction essay *How the Poor Die* (1946). The latter stands as a definitive, blow-by-blow account of the treatment he received during his two-week spell at L'Hôpital Cochin.[2]

HOW THE POOR DIE

L'Hôpital Cochin offered Orwell nothing short of torture. Upon arrival, he was met with an aggressive and unpleasant interrogation by the hospital's receptionist – lasting a full twenty minutes and which, given his feverish temperature of 'around about' 103 degrees Fahrenheit,[3] tested his ability to stay conscious.[4] Next, Orwell was given a hot bath: 'a compulsory routine for all newcomers, apparently, just as in prison or the workhouse'.[5]

His clothes were stowed and replaced with the hospital's uniform of a linen nightshirt and blue dressing gown. In this scanty clothing, he was led barefoot through the open air – on a brisk February evening, and with suspected pneumonia – to the main hospital building. Inside, dim light illuminated rows of beds, each just a few inches, and a 'foul smell, faecal and yet sweetish' filled his nose.

Orwell was humiliated, disgusted and frightened on the ward. The experience led him to conclude that there is a substantial difference between how the poor and the rich die:

> In the public wards of a hospital you see horrors that you don't seem to meet with among people who manage to die in their own homes, as though certain diseases only attack people at the lower income levels.[6]

The most affluent of Orwell's contemporaries could expect to expire in relative comfort. Most of them would pay for a doctor to deliver care in their own home. If they did need to visit hospital, they would book a private room – with better care, nicer food, more focused attention, in short: more dignity. The poor could expect a far more brutal, undignified and painful experience in tightly packed wards. The institution of the hospital, for them, was of the same genre as the prison block or the torture chamber.

Orwell's story is not just about France. It's not pure travel writing, nor is it designed to simply make his British readers grateful for what they have by comparison. Rather, it's a story that epitomises the growing demands in the 1940s for major improvements to the country's health system, and which captures the growing public distaste for the health inequalities present in mid-twentieth century Britain.[7]

It was within this context that the country elected the radical Attlee government, promising a system of universal healthcare. After a long and contested legislative process, the National Health Service was born on 5 July 1948 – with the explicit objective of providing everyone with the healthcare they needed: regardless of class status, income, religion, home address, or place of birth. It was meant, once and for all, to solve the kind of injustices about which Orwell had written.

THE GREAT EQUALISER

The sheer existence of the NHS gives rise to a pervasive idea today that we are all equal in the face of disease. This was certainly an idea that commentators looked to push in the early stages of Covid-19.

The Sunday Express published an official leader to this effect on March 15 2020.[8] In the same month, John Harris wrote in the *Guardian* that 'Coronavirus means we really are, finally, all in this together'.[9] In between the two, the *Evening Standard* declared that 'London Stands Together'.[10]

Madonna, broadcasting from a marble bathtub sprinkled with rose petals, recorded a video message calling the virus 'the great equaliser'.[11]

The actual experience of Covid couldn't be in starker contrast to these early proclamations. The disparities became clear from the moment we first learned the identities of the people dying from the disease. The national media took particular interest in the fate of NHS workers. And as they began to contract the virus, and tragically began to die, it was not uncommon to see their faces lined up on the front pages of the morning papers. Displayed in this way, something became clear: very few of the faces were white.

On 2 June 2020, anecdote was backed by evidence when Public Health England (PHE) published data on the pandemic's inequalities.[12] Compared to previous years, excess deaths among white men had doubled. But among Asian men, they had tripled. And among Black men, they had quadrupled.[13] The report found similar patterns of mortality by ethnicity among women as well.

The same PHE report also implicated class in Covid's injustices, and subsequent data has revealed this relationship yet more clearly. Official statistics now show the occupations with the highest Covid-19 mortality rates in 2020 were, in descending order: bakers, publicans, butchers, police officers, vehicle valets and cleaners, restaurant managers, hairdressers, care workers and home carers, metal working machine operatives, bank clerks, food and drink process operatives, chefs, taxi drivers and chauffeurs, security guards, roofers, waiters, ambulance staff, nursing assistants, catering and bar managers, hospital porters, caterers, and nurses.[14] Every occupation on this list had a Covid mortality rate at least double the average (and as much as twenty times larger).[15] And the clear pattern is that these most vulnerable professional groups predominantly fill jobs that are low paid and unable to offer work from home, but which are vital to maintaining the country.

'Long Covid' – a particularly serious form of the virus, with as many as 200 symptoms according to researchers at University College London[16] – has a similar epidemiology. According to estimates from the Office for National Statistics (ONS), about a million people in the UK had long Covid as of July 2021.[17] Of that million, health and care workers, people aged 35 to 69, women and those with a disability made up a disproportionate number of cases.[18] Moreover, people living in the most deprived parts of the country – a measure obviously related to class and occupation – were also more likely to report having long Covid at the time of the analysis.

So strong is the link between job, class and long Covid, that there have been calls for the illness to be categorised as an 'occupational disease' – to ensure sufferers are eligible for Industrial Injuries Disablement Benefit (IIDB) payments.[19] Despite this, there has been little in terms of recognition, support, or compensation.

INJUSTICE AT SCALE

Severe health disparities are not unique to the pandemic. In fact, the inequalities observed run along the same lines as health injustice before it. Recent estimates put life expectancy for men in the most deprived parts of the country at nearly ten years less than those in the least deprived. Among women, the gap is 7.6 years. The inequality in healthy life expectancy[20] was twice as high – 19.0 years for men and 19.3 years for women.[21] Compared to people in the least deprived parts of the country, those living in the most deprived communities are two times more likely to be diagnosed with lung cancer, and 1.5 times more likely to be diagnosed with prostate cancer.[22] Similar figures can be found for almost every major physical and mental health condition.

That means that while Covid-19 was defined by inequality, and enacted injustice at massive scale, it was not the pandemic that put the conditions in place for this injustice. Covid simply exposed and exploited the existing structural vulnerabilities in the country's health system. The conclusion we must level with is that despite the landmark democratic socialist achievement of a National Health Service in 1948 – and the work done since to solidify and protect those gains – we still have a public health system that disproportionately distributes good health to the wealthy and the powerful, and poor health to the poorest and most marginalised.

It is the same status quo that Orwell and others were railing against, and which was seen to justify radical change, over seven decades ago.

*   *   *

Injustice wasn't the only metric through which the Covid pandemic exposed that something isn't quite right with our public health system's status quo. The UK's overall pandemic outcomes also testify to that fact.

In February 2021, as our vaccine programme began to pick up pace, the UK had experienced 1 in every 25 Covid deaths globally, despite being home to just 1 in every 100 people alive on Earth.[23] Even then, the Covid death count was only suppressed by the withdrawal of universal care elsewhere in the health system. Millions of appointments were cancelled, from routine operations to cancer treatments.

Research published in the spring of 2021 by the Institute for Public Policy Research (IPPR) showed both the extent of this disruption, and the consequences it could have on healthcare in years to come. England lost a decade of progress on cardiovascular disease outcomes, thanks to 5,500 'excess' deaths in 2020. It can expect a further 12,000 cases of heart and attack and stroke over the next five years because of the pandemic.[24] As much as a decade of progress on five-year cancer survival was lost, too, with thousands of extra deaths from cancer now expected from disruptions to screening, referrals and treatment.[25] Elsewhere, checks on people with the most severe mental illnesses fell a third below their target level. Eating disorder referrals amongst children doubled, while treatment waiting lists reached new, five-year highs in 2020/1.[26] Overall, and at the time of writing, the pandemic is expected to create an extra 1.8 million mental health referrals, piling pressure on an already stretched part of the system.[27]

The blame doesn't lie with the individual people of this country. News pages have been filled by pictures of panic buying, empty shelves, packed tube carriages and overflowing beaches. But harder evidence often tells a different story – a British people who were often remarkable for their pandemic solidarity. Most did stay home. The *University College London Covid-19 Social Study*, which followed 70,000 participants over a sustained period, found consistently high compliance with Covid-19 rules – including levels of up to 90 per cent in December 2020 and 96 per cent in January 2021.[28] Mutual aid groups also sprung up across the country.[29] Solidarity funds were set up to help people get through tough times. People made protective gear for NHS workers and came out to clap on Thursday evenings.

The failure is not about individual responsibility. Rather, it's entirely about flaws with our public health system and institutions. Just as in the 1940s, it is evident that massive disruption and destruction must be followed by radical thinking and a bold vision for change.

CRISIS AND CHANGE

Crisis is perhaps the key enabler of change. In the *Communist Manifesto*, Karl Marx and Fredrich Engels describe how:

> a society that has conjured up such gigantic means of production and of exchange is like the sorcerer who is no longer able to control the powers of the nether world whom he has called up by his spells.[30]

Here, the authors refer to a predilection to crisis innate in capitalism. It is an observation often paraphrased as the 'boom and bust cycle' today – a flaw which no capitalist economy has ever been able to resolve. Their final argument is that production will push capitalism into ever greater crises – any one of which could lead to its ultimate destruction.

Milton Friedman agrees on the political significance of crises:

> Only a crisis – actual or perceived – produces real change. When that crisis occurs, the actions that are taken depend on the ideas that are lying around. That, I believe, is our basic function: to develop alternatives to existing policies, to keep them alive and available until the politically impossible becomes politically inevitable.[31]

For Friedman, a crisis makes change possible, but the definition of that change will depend on who wins the subsequent battle of ideas. Elsewhere, various writers, politicians and policy thinkers – William Beveridge, Barack Obama, John Kingdon, Winston Churchill and Rosa Luxemburg among them – have subscribed to the idea of crisis as an engine of radical change.

As crises go, the pandemic is evidently big enough to lead to fundamental change. Covid has had the economic impact of a credit crunch, the human impact of a world war and the societal impact of an industrial revolution. As of March 2021, in the UK, it had killed 125,000 people,[32] caused GDP to decline by 10 per cent[33] and closed schools and workplaces, forcing many to go more than a year without seeing their loved ones. Its magnitude cannot be overstated.

The question is who is best prepared to steer the direction of change when it comes. The thinkers I've referenced, who see crisis as a vehicle for change, subscribe to very different politics. That means the change springing forth from Covid will not be uncontested. Instead, it will come down to a competition of different viewpoints from across the political spectrum – with each looking to define the form our society will take in the aftermath of this epoch-defining event.

We only need to look at 2008 and the aftermath of the global financial crash to see that this is true. As much as the left were emboldened in the subsequent decade, often in bolder and decentralised activism and campaigns, so too were the right. Many countries experienced a significant shift to the right, including dangerous and ongoing lurches towards fascism.[34] Jobbik entered government in Hungary, as did the Lega Nord in Italy. Austria's Freedom Party, Switzerland's People's Party, Denmark's People's Party, Belgium's New Flemish Alliance, Poland's PiS (Law and Justice) and France's National Front[35] are all populist or far-right parties that recorded vote shares of 20 per cent or more at a national election within the last decade.

This is not unique to the financial crash. A 2016 study showed that political polarisation regularly follows crises of this type and severity.[36] In terms of pandemics, analysis has linked major infectious disease episodes to shifts to right-wing populism – including links between Spanish Flu mortality and support for the Nazi party in Germany[37] – but also to revolutions by workers and other marginalised groups: the peasant revolt (fourteenth century England),[38] the 1830 and 1848 uprisings (France),[39] and the riots in Russia that pre-empted and supported the Russian Revolution.[40]

The change coming out of Covid could be radical and just. It could create a better public health system, that distributes good health, more justly, to the people who need it. But we must also take seriously the threat that it could be regressive, or simply magnify the problems that exist within the current status quo. We stand then at a crossroads: in need of ideas, strategy and momentum.

CAN THE LEFT WIN?

Contemporary health movements and activism have remarkable energy. In 2018, I joined a march to Downing Street called 'March for the NHS'. The atmosphere was eclectic. Tens of thousands of people had taken to the streets, to journey through central London and demand better health. The calls were simple: more money in the NHS, better treatment for health workers and – most of all – private providers kicked out from the system. The march was a demonstration of the sheer passion and energy health inspires. Hours before the set start time, there were impromptu platforms with speakers addressing small crowds of activists. 'Who's NHS? Our NHS!', rang out through the crowd.

There is a reason that health inspires passion on a scale few other agendas do. People care about it for its own sake, and as a site of wider social justice. It is seen as integral to the society we've built, a canary in the coal mine for fairness in our country. The idea of people dying because they didn't have the means to pay for treatment is one of the most abhorrent to our collective imagination.

I admire this. It's one of the reasons I work in health. Nonetheless, there are grounds for stepping back to take a constructive look at the strategy through which the left's movement – the thinkers, politicians, researchers, campaigners, journalists, commentators, filmmakers, social media activists and diversity of people who subscribe to its values – approach the agenda.

There is one analogy that particularly helps us to understand its general nature. The aggregate approach to health in the left movement is reminiscent of how Troy approached its city defences. The NHS has become *the* citadel of democratic socialism, built in 1948 and standing ever since. The left's role has become defined explicitly by strengthening those defences and fortifying the perimeter, in anticipation of ideological assault. We are stuck in a rear-guard action.

That is to say, when it comes to health, our movements, politicians, journalists, thinkers and activists often embody what I define as a fundamentally defensive approach. In simple terms, the logic works as follows. We believe in 1948 as an ultimate victory for the left on the health agenda. The National Health Service, formed by Bevan, is proof that democratic socialist principles can work and that they do make people's lives better. The leftist strategy in health has therefore become defined by maintaining the status quo. If the NHS is democratic socialism in action, then our mission is to protect that from annihilation.

Perhaps it is easiest to define it in terms of what we defend it against. There are a number of perceived threats to 'our NHS': pay cuts, funding cuts and local hospital closures among them. But by far the most oft-cited threat to is the idea of the **sell-off**. Whether in a quick shock-and-awe victory (e.g., an American trade deal) or a more gradual process, the defensive approach is preoccupied with a perpetual threat of the NHS's imminent destruction though some form of mass privatisation. Other issues, from funding cuts to pay-for-service reconfiguration, are often themselves brought back to this primary focal point.

There is, of course, merit in opposing privatisation. Arguments that it is a) not really a risk at all, or that b) it would somehow improve the NHS, are incoherent with the evidence. The former argument has been challenged by the pandemic, which will almost certainly increase the role of the private sector in UK healthcare. As Covid-19 shocked the NHS and stretched its capacity in 2020, the private sector seemed to offer an initial hand of comfort. For example, at the peak of the crisis, independent sector capacity was offered to the NHS at cost price. Yet, we must question the purity of motives when a leaked email from the chief executive of Serco – Rupert Soames – talked of collaboration as little more than a way to 'cement the position of the private sector' in the NHS's supply chain.[41] The message recasts 'generosity' as an attempt to build dependency, with an intention to then exploit.

The latter argument, meanwhile, has been put to bed by systematic review: for example, as published in the *British Medical Journal* by Neena Modi and her colleagues in 2018.[42] Their work shows, first, that private healthcare provision is not efficient: normally, a key argument in its favour. Instead, public hospitals tend to demonstrate either equal or greater efficiency than their private counterparts.[43] Second, they highlight a private sector tendency towards 'cherry picking' their patients – essentially, when allowed to be part of a mixed-economy healthcare model, it scoops up the simplest, richest (i.e. most profitable) patients and leaves the public sector with the most complicated, chronic cases.[44] Finally, they highlight that private companies tend to avoid scrutiny: in the search for a good reputation, few private providers are willing to undertake quite the level of auditing that public bodies undergo.

Despite this, the government has indicated that they are happy to allow the private sector a greater role in the supply chain in the years to come. Rather than provide significant public capacity to get through the post-Covid backlog, the NHS is being forced to procure significant amounts of private capacity. As *the Health Service Journal*, one of the sector's most respected media outlets, discovered in October 2020, private providers have been asked to apply to provide £10bn worth of NHS services over the next four years.[45] This represents a one-off shift to the private sector worth around 0.2 per cent of the annual NHS budget – and though that might not sound like a lot, it is not hard for these kinds of increments to make up a large proportion of the whole.

Even so, a slight increase remains more likely than a wholescale takeover by the private sector. Analysis by the Nuffield Trust indicates there have been two big jumps in the proportion of NHS spend going to the private sector this century. The first was due to New Labour's introduction of independent sector treatment providers and the second came after the market-orientated Health and Social Care Act in 2012.[46] But it is equally true that 70 per cent of the NHS private spend are things that are not often politically contested. The fact is that GPs, dentists and optometrists are private sector remains by far the greatest source of privatisation in the NHS – suggesting the left has been broadly successful in preventing further, major source of privatisation from emerging in the last seven decades.

THE PROBLEM WITH DEFENCE

Evidently there is some danger ahead, but my critique isn't about our opposition to privatisation per se. Rather, it is that the left's movement has focused on defence far too exclusively. In our rear-guard action against the wrecking ball of privatisation, we have arguably forgotten about the other things that matter. And should we find ourselves unable to rectify that, to balance defending what is good about the NHS with a transformative imagination about what a radically better public health system could look like, we will both fail to solve the defining challenges in health today and leave ourselves vulnerable to major problems in the future.

The problem with a rear-guard action is that, by definition, it is interested in protecting the status quo. This leads us to two, critical oversights. The first is an existential threat that could equally destroy the NHS, within decades, should it simply remain in stasis: the spectre of the **buyout**. As much as privatisation and a 'sell-off' would prove destructive, there is equal risk posed by people abandoning the NHS for insurance schemes or direct payment options. If we spend too much time protecting the way things are, and not enough time developing a vision for a genuinely brilliant NHS, we will allow this to happen without adequate scrutiny or opposition.

The second oversight is the limit on how effective and fair a public health and care system we can achieve while only focusing on the NHS. Good health, just health, sustainable health: all rely on the totality of our public health system, in which the NHS is just one part. But a defensive approach predisposes us to overly focus on the NHS ('NHS-centrism'). If the NHS remains the limit of our health horizons, alongside perhaps some limited local authority-run health services, we will miss the opportunity to put forward a genuinely holistic and transformative vision for what good health really means.

THE BUYOUT

Public ownership was a key founding principle of the NHS. But the biggest threat to the health service today isn't an end to public ownership.[47] It is an all-out assault of the extent of its universality.

Nye Bevan understood that the viability of the NHS relied, first and foremost, on keeping performance at the 'frontier' of what is possible. As such, 'Universalising the Best' was integral to his vision, as he told the House of Commons at the second reading of his NHS Bill:

> [. . .] our intention [is] that we should universalise the best, [so] that we shall promise every citizen in this country the same standard of service.[48]

It is a less well-remembered and less oft-cited phrase today, but it is crucial.

What Bevan recognised was that anything less than the most comprehensive health service provides those who can afford it with an incentive to 'buy-out'. That is, it gives them a reason to supplement or replace their public entitlement to healthcare with private health services and insurance – to skip long waiting lists, access novel treatments, receive better technology and digital tools, become eligible for clinical trials, or even to travel to other countries to receive their treatment.[49] The bigger the gap between what the NHS could provide and what it does provide, the stronger the incentive to buy-out – and the larger the group that is incentivised to do so.

The data shows that this is happening. The number of people using private insurance to avoid waiting times is on the rise. In January 2021, market analysts LaingBuisson released a study showing that the total amount spent on private hospital surgery had reached £1.1 billion in value, according to the latest data.[50] That's a 7.4 per cent increase in the self-paying market. A further edition of the research, released in April 2021, showed confidence that there would be further growth in the years to come – with the 4.5 million patients waiting for planned NHS care (as of December 2020) a key driver.[51]

This follows 2017 research by Intuition Communications, which found that profit-driven hospital firms were experiencing a 15 to 25 per cent rise in 'self-payers' funding their own care.[52] And in 2020, Compare the Market – the insurance price comparison website – reported a 40 per cent increase in health insurance sales, compared to 2019, as people looked to insulate themselves against the waiting time increases being brought about by Covid-19.[53]

This fits as part of a longer-term shift. In the 1970s, the UK was the country that used general taxation to fund the greatest proportion of its health services.[54] Yet by 1996, the UK was the advanced economy with the fastest growing shift to 'out of pocket' payments. Where this had accounted for just a tiny proportion of total health spend in 1980 – equal to 0.46 per cent of GDP (value of around $2.5 billion), by 1997 it was equivalent to almost 1.3 per cent of UK GDP (value of around $20 billion).[55] After a small relative drop between 2002 and 2006, the use of out-of-pocket payments to fund health continued its rise – reaching nearly 1.8 per cent of GDP in 2020 (value of around $50 billion). Overall, that's a massive increase in healthcare spend coming from individual, private bank accounts over the last four decades.[56]

A crucial difference between the buy-out and the sell-off is that the former does not need the NHS to be sold, or its budget to be cut. It simply needs public health investment to lag behind the sum of growing need and advancing innovation – that is, to remain in stasis. It is a method of transitioning from comprehensive service to a string-bare safety net that requires little to no expenditure of political capital by the right.

The state of dentistry serves as a warning of the risks this kind of long-term trend poses. In Bevan's original conception, dentistry was within the NHS. The use of charges was introduced in 1951[57] (for dentures) and expanded in 1952.[58] Slowly, over time, charges have risen – with a particularly major acceleration in 1992. As a result, a crisis of access has emerged, and the number of people going to the dentist has steadily dropped.[59] In the place of professional dentistry home dentistry returned. Gut-wrenching stories have become common – of people using pliers to extract teeth or people filling their teeth with Polyfilla and other hardware store products.[60] It's a micro-example of what can happen when we acclimatise ourselves to topping-up our care and allowing the NHS to become an ever-more limited safety net – rather than a method through which we collectively buy the best possible healthcare for everyone.

The existential threat would come in the form of weakened electoral support. There has always been strong public consensus against cuts to the NHS – a service that has provided the best for 95 per cent of the population at a lower cost in tax than they would pay in a market-based private model. This popularity contrasts with the fragility of public support for state benefits – particularly cash benefits for the unemployed. Since the British Social Attitudes survey first began in the 1980s, support for higher welfare payments has oscillated significantly – including sustained periods of support for cutting provision, and more recent support for increasing provision.[61] That instability is markedly different to the consistency of support shown for our NHS – support that sustains its existence.

In the end, it might seem like the buy-out and the sell-off aren't that different. They both end with a conditional NHS, run for profit and unfit for purpose. But we should be far more worried about the buy-out, for three key reasons. First, it is stealthier, and far less costly for the right to implement. Second, it is even more brutally unequal. And lastly, it is a route to reversing the humanising achievements of the NHS – and one for which the left is fundamentally unprepared.

We also need to recognise that reacting to the buy-out requires a very different movement. A rear-guard action makes sense if the threat is a 'big bang'-style sale of the NHS, through either a Thatcher-esque denationalisation process or an American trade deal. But defensive approaches are implicitly about maintaining stasis and supporting the status quo, and that just won't work against the sell-off. Instead, we will need to avoid the space between what health and care the state *could* theoretically provide, and what health and care it *does* provide, from growing. That means having a compelling, radical and transformative health vision for the future – which is not something defensive activism can provide. As such, it is critical to the future of our health and our health institutions that we're able to move onto the offensive, and to articulate a conception of universalising the best fit for the twenty-first century.

NHS CENTRISM: LOOKING BEYOND 'OUR NHS'

Even then, a vision that only focuses on the NHS will not be nearly enough to secure and sustain health justice. NHS-centrism is implicit in any conception of 'defending the NHS'. Yet, the biggest emerging heath and care challenges demand that we look beyond our beloved National Health Service.

In the last 75 years, we have seen a fundamental shift in the country's health needs. The transition can be shown by comparing the big causes of mortality in the two periods. In the 1940s, heart disease and strokes killed 4 in 10 people – often suddenly. Tuberculosis still killed 1 in 20. Infant mortality was nearly ten times higher than it is today.[62] Polio and diphtheria remained prevalent. It was a period when coronary heart disease killed 166,000 in Britain – more than twice as many as the circa 60,000 today (despite substantial population growth since then).[63]

The change since has been defined by three main trends. First, there has been the rise in the age of the UK population, from around 5 million people aged 65 and older in 1948, to 12.5 million people aged 65 or older in 2020. This means the average individual now has more ill-health. Second, a significant rise in long-term chronic health conditions – Type II diabetes, asthma, arthritis and some forms of dementia. Third, the fact that many diseases that presented as acute in the 1940s are taking on a more chronic profile. In 1970, someone could expect to live one year from the point of receiving their cancer diagnosis: today they can expect to live up to six years.[64]

If a rise in chronic conditions has defined the change in health needs over the last fifty years, health in the first half of the twenty-first century will be defined by the challenges posed by 'multiple conditions'.[65] Today, around one in four adults have two or more health conditions – equating to around 14.2 million people in England.[66] People with multiple conditions make up 55 per cent of NHS costs for hospital admissions and outpatient visits. And in the most deprived parts of the country, the average age of someone with multiple conditions is 61 – but lower life expectancy means that they can also expect to live with them for 12 to 17 years.[67]

These statistics all feed into one of the greatest health and care challenges we face: the growing gap between how long we can expect to live overall, and how long we can expect to live with a 'reasonable' level of health. While healthy life expectancy has risen in the last century, it has not risen nearly as fast as life expectancy. On average, someone can now expect to live as much as 15 to 20 years of their life in below 'reasonable' quality health.[68] That means we are spending an ever-greater proportion of our lives in poor health – on average, the entirety of our retirement.

Stalling longevity is also a worry. In many parts of the country, life expectancy was stagnant or regressing before the pandemic[69] – in many cases, due to factors over which the NHS has little control. In a major 2020 review, Professor Sir Michael Marmot implicated child poverty, variation in employment, experience of fuel poverty, food poverty and poverty, rising household debt and the rise of poor housing as the key factors.[70] Other research has implicated obesity.[71] And a similar stall or even an emerging reversal in life expectancy in America has been linked to rising 'deaths of despair' – a now well-established rise in death at middle age amongst people without BA degrees, linked to opioids, other drug abuse, alcohol-related diseases and suicide.[72]

The NHS is best placed to deal with exactly none of these trends and future challenges. It is designed only to pick up the pieces.

For the sake of our health today and in the future, we need to radically reimagine what our public health system can look like. The reality of stalling life expectancy, multiple chronic conditions and an ageing population are more than a treatment service, as one arm of the welfare state, can cope with. Instead, they demand we build a health system that prevents illness, promotes health at every turn, that ensures good lives for people living with chronic illnesses or disabilities. That does not mean hospitals become irrelevant, or that the left needs to become anti-NHS. Rather, it will mean we need to extend our ideals outside of the brick-and-mortar NHS – into communities, into social policy, into our economic models.

The pandemic has added urgency to that mission. It was underlying health conditions – a great many of which could have been prevented by pre-emptive social interventions – that drove vulnerability to the virus. It was occupation, sick pay, access to furlough and wealth inequality that defined whether people could bunker down in their rural second homes or had to work as usual through the pandemic. Covid has underscored the need to view public health as a cohesive, distributive system – in which we proactively increase the total stock of health in the country, and then ensure it is distributed fairly.

With all that said, it is worrying that there are many examples where Covid-19 has catalysed a greater and more explicit focus on the NHS, rather than a broader focus on the whole public health system. One indicative example that has gained traction is the 'NHS New Deal'. At the time of writing, the website for the campaign contends:

For more than 70 years the NHS has cared for us. It's there for us when we need it most. But politicians have continually mistreated the NHS. And during the pandemic, it has come close to collapse. Now we have a plan to win a New Deal for the NHS. This will mean proper funding for our NHS. Support for Doctors and Nurses to do their jobs. Putting the health of patients above the interests of big corporations. Tackling inequalities so that all of us get the healthcare we need and deserve. Our NHS needs you. Last year millions of us clapped for key workers and painted rainbows in our windows. Now we need to turn that support into action.[73]

The copy itself is very hard to disagree with. In fact, it's admirable. But it is also typical of the marginalisation of the rest of the public health and care system from the left's health activism. Until these aspects are mainstreamed in the most developed, most well-funded and most visible parts of the movement, it will be very hard to deliver the kind of advances the post-pandemic world needs.

THE FIVE FRONTIERS

This book is about the health frontiers that span out before us. Based on a decade of research, I have mapped out five frontiers where there are the biggest opportunities to drive forward health improvement and health justice. Some of these frontiers are about reinventing existing institutions and services. Others are about expanding the principles from the NHS into bold new agendas.

The frontiers provide the structure of the book, with each the focus of a chapter. They are put forward as a foundation for a more strategic social movement, one more informed by the future realities and challenges of our population's health.

The inclusion of each frontier is guided by this book's twin aims: maximising the stock of the nation's health, and making the distribution of good health more just. As such, each chapter is designed to stand alone – in putting forward evidence, establishing problems and suggesting transformative new ideas. But each chapter is also designed to fit together into a larger vision: a cohesive new blueprint for better health.

Chapter One begins with the **NHS frontier**. The NHS comes first intentionally. It's an opportunity to dive more deeply into the discourses that underpin the left's defensive strategy and look, in more depth, at how this approach works in practice. I ask whether these narratives are serving us, our health and our health service in the best possible way. And I put forward an alternative – based on the concept of addressing the most pressing issues undermining universal care and based on conceptualising Universalise the Best as a focal point of our movement.

Chapter Two looks at the **Social Justice Frontier**. It begins to define what I mean, practically, by distributive public health. I argue that we need an expansion of Bevan's principles from medical to social interventions – through a new Universal Public Health Service. Fundamentally, this chapter argues we need to be as willing to prevent a health need by giving someone a state funded home, as we are to treat a health need by giving someone a state funded course of chemotherapy.

Chapter Three covers the **Economic Frontier**. It argues that health exploitation by profit-driven corporations is rife. Yet, too often, critiques of this reality are limited by a focus on individual businesses and sectors – rather than a genuine understanding of how this is enabled, incentivised, and normalised by our dominant economic model. I outline the case for a Public Health Net Zero – as a tool to fundamentally change the relationship between health and wealth – and to better protect health from the interests of capital

Chapter Four explores the **Care Frontier**. Care is one of the areas where grassroots and left movements have begun, in places, to expand their horizons. However, while there are some very good proposals, we have stopped short of truly transformative thinking. If today's care homes are the modern equivalent of the twentieth century's asylums, then our policies simply make the asylums free – they do not tear them down. We need to use the foundations of consensus to build a vision not only of how social care provision works, but what social care is, does, looks like and prioritises.

Chapter Five finishes with the **Sustainability Frontier**. It would be easy for the pandemic to make our approach to health more insular, more nativist. On the right, this might come from a greater focus on 'security' – a paradigm that is nationalistic and border-focused. Among the left's movement, it might come from an even more narrow focus on the NHS and outsourcing. This is incongruent with the continuing rise in global health vulnerability – and this chapter argues we need to both comprehend the urgency of the wider health context, and to build a vision for how the UK should now react.

The final chapter brings the frontiers together and explores the case for the Public Health New Deal. I consider how well the interventions fit together. I address key questions such as whether we can afford them, at what scale would we deliver them, and whether we can really prevent privatisation without focusing on it as explicitly.

The shock of war and inexcusable levels of health inequality combined to create the conditions for the NHS in 1948. After the shock of Covid, and in the face of huge health uncertainty and injustice today, the time for radical public health policy has come once again.

OUR HEALTH: A RADICAL NEW BLUEPRINT

1. **The NHS**: A new 'Universalise the Best' mission in the NHS, replacing decades of toxic New Public Management (Chapter 1)
2. **Social Justice**: A Universal Public Health Service, meeting health need long before a diagnosis (Chapter 2)
3. **Economy**: A public health net zero target overseen by a new public health unit, to end health exploitation by capital (Chapter 3)
4. **Social Care**: Expansion of National Care Service concept to cover what care is for, not just how care is provided and procured (Chapter 4)
5. **Sustainability**: UK policy that supports global health sustainability and promises future generations a legacy of better health (Chapter 5)

1
The NHS Frontier

It might seem strange, in a book that has just critiqued the NHS-centrism of much contemporary health activism, to begin by considering the NHS. However, as the institution so explicitly central to how the left approaches health, beginning here provides an opportunity to understand our movement a little better.

If our mainstream narrative can be said to have a common thread, it's Romanticism. The stories our movement tells often rest on a common foundation of the idyll, the emotive, the nostalgic. Our version of barricading the NHS is putting it forward in an idealised form – both to highlight what is right about our politics, and to protect the institution from smear and attack. It is the mechanism we have developed, on the left, to protect and conserve the status quo on an agenda where we believe we have won the argument.

Examples of Romanticism are not hard to find within the Labour Party. One illustrative example comes from Nick Thomas-Symonds' book *Nye: The Political Life of Aneurin Bevan*:[1]

> The National Health Service that he created on 5 July 1948 is no mere monument to his success. Rather, it is a living, breathing example of his democratic-socialist principles, applied pragmatically to bring a better life for his fellow citizens. With a budget of over £108 billion, the modern-day NHS is the world's largest publicly funded health service, employing more than 1.7 million people and providing healthcare to over 63 million people in the UK. Such is the scale of Bevan's achievement that the central principle of the NHS, care free at the point of delivery on the basis of need regardless of wealth, is uncontested by any major political party over 60 years after the service's foundation.[2]

Elsewhere, the story juxtaposes Romanticism of the NHS against the reality of an imminent, existential threat. This was the story told in the 2019 Labour Party election manifesto:

The National health Service is one of Labour's proudest achievements. The right to free-at-the-point-of-use healthcare, universal and comprehensive in scope, is socialism in action . . . [But] A decade of Tory health cuts and privatisations has pushed our greatest institution to the brink.[3]

The manifesto text was brought to life on 27 November, 2019, when the then Leader of the Opposition Jeremy Corbyn convened a major press conference to reveal official documents that purported to show the NHS was 'on the table' in any US trade deal.

In fact, the twinned combination of narratives describing the 'NHS as our proudest achievement' and the NHS as at risk of 'imminent destruction' has defined the party's modern election platform. It's a narrative that brings together Blair and Kinnock, Miliband and Corbyn, Harold Wilson and Hugh Gaitskell. Though the Labour Party's vision and leadership in 1997 and 2017 seem almost irreconcilable, both released final press releases with the same headline: '24 hours to [vote Labour and] save the NHS'.[4]

A Romantic discourse is not exclusive to Westminster. At the opening ceremony of the 2012 London Olympics, director Danny Boyle paid homage to the National Health Service. Set to the music of Mike Oldfield, dancers depicted staff and patients – all set within one of the NHS's most famous institutions: The Great Ormond Street Hospital.

The scene showed little of the realities of healthcare. The hospitals were glisteningly clean. The uniforms were crisp and pressed. The nurses and doctors were numerous and well rested. The child patients were jumping, happily, on their beds. But then, the point of the dance wasn't to give a realist account of the reality of illness or healthcare work. It wasn't Orwell's *How the Poor Die*.

Instead, Boyle's portrayal of the NHS is all to do with the health service as a symbol. The NHS functions as a signifier of our country's progressive capability – our capacity for kindness, our solidarity with our fellow people, our compassion for those in need. Team GB later described the scene as: 'Togetherness, compassion, spirit and support. The NHS embodies everything that is great about our society'.[5]

The Romantic and defensive qualities of the performance were not lost on its audience. Broadcaster Steve Richards, writing in *The Independent*, concluded that:

As the NHS was celebrated vividly with bright lights and hundreds of dancing nurses, I was reminded of *Hamlet*, the scene when Hamlet asks the players to act out his father's murder . . . At the opening ceremony, David Cameron must have felt a little like Claudius as he watched Danny Boyle's players: a Prime Minister who seeks to overhaul the NHS . . . watching a jubilant portrayal of the NHS as it is and was.[6]

That is, he argues that the Olympic ceremony juxtaposed its vision of the NHS against the Health Secretary Andrew Lansley's 2012 Health and Social Care Act – a piece of legislation many viewed as a certain route to massive privatisation.[7]

HEROES

The association of NHS and heroism was by no means unheard of before 2020 – but usage of 'hero' in the same breath as 'NHS' exploded as the Covid-19 pandemic took hold in mid-March. It is hard to pin-point an exact origin, or whether it was steered more from the right or the left. Early articles in media associated with both the right and the left used this framing extensively from around 17 March, as hospitals began to feel significant pressure – and a week before the Prime Minister gave the first 'stay at home' order. Equally, Hansard registers record use of the association spontaneously across parties. The earliest adopters in the Commons registers include Jeremy Corbyn, John McDonnell (Labour) and Ian Blackford (SNP).

Early on, the right's discourse was more likely to be defined by war rhetoric – epitomised in early Covid-19 briefings by Boris Johnson and, in the US, Donald Trump.[8] By contrast, heroism in the NHS has gone on to become the dominant aspect of left pandemic discourse – an image evoked regularly, whether in answer to the poor provision of PPE in Spring 2020 or the government's offer of a 1 per cent NHS pay rise in Spring 2021.

In reaction to the latter, trade union GMB's pay justice campaign called on the government to 'give our NHS heroes a proper pay increase'; The Labour Party promised to 'fight for a significant real-terms pay increase for NHS Covid heroes';[9] The Liberal Democrats 'slammed' the offer of 1 per cent pay rise as an 'insult to our NHS heroes';[10] *The Mirror* ran with headlines like 'NHS heroes take to the streets to demand a pay rise from Tory Ministers'.[11]

There is absolutely no doubt that NHS workers have done remarkable work, at huge personal cost, during Covid-19. Neither does it contradict that reality to suggest 'hero' is a classic trope of Romantic discourse – and one that is not entirely unproblematic. As has been pointed out by frontline workers themselves, heroism suggests a certain sense of infallibility – workers who find strength to persevere, despite overwhelming obstacles. But the reality is NHS workers are human: they feel pain, they have flaws, they get things wrong sometimes and they burn-out if they're pushed too hard.[12] 'Hero' sets a standard of exceptionalism that workers themselves have not always found helpful or healthy.

The hero trope is familiar from its use during times of war – particularly, in propaganda designed to encourage young, working-class men to give their lives for their country on foreign fields. It inspired Wilfred Owen's poem *Dulce et Decorum Est*, in 1918:

If in some smothering dreams, you too could pace
Behind the wagon that we flung him in,
And watch the white eyes writhing in his face,
His hanging face, like a devil's sick of sin;
[. . .]
My friend, you would not tell with such high zest
To children ardent for some desperate glory,
The old Lie: *Dulce et decorum est*
Pro patria mori.[13]

The Romanticism of heroism, Owen suggests, ignores the horrors and pains of war, and poorly serves the soldiers who fight in them. Similarly, we must ask if the Romantic, defensive approach we're employing is genuinely serving our NHS and the people who run it.

EXPLORING THE EVIDENCE

Since 2009, the polling company YouGov have tracked the British public's perceptions of NHS performance in comparison to its international peers. At the start of the period, only about one in seven respondents thought that the NHS performed less well than other health systems – while one in three thought it was better.[14] By April 2021, after more than a year of Covid – and as newspaper headlines warned of record waiting times and disrupted cancer care – the number of people who thought the

NHS was the world's best had actually increased. Just one in ten people now thought it performed less well than comparators (down six points), while 42 per cent of people thought it was better (up nine points).[15]

On their own, public attitudes don't really tell us much about whether the NHS *is* the world's best health system. The nuances of the French, German, Singaporean or Canadian systems are not common conversations in the nation's pubs, restaurants, or dinner tables – and few of us have a direct basis for such a comparison. What public attitudes data show is not evidence that the NHS *is the best*, only that the public believe it is.

The study most often used to back up this belief comes from the American foundation the Commonwealth Fund. In their 2017 global rankings, the NHS came top against health systems from 11 advanced economies.[16] That enviable position was thanks to excellent scores for care processes, levels of equity, levels of access and administrative efficiency.[17] The NHS did comparatively poorly in just one area: it comes second bottom on healthcare outcomes.[18]

It sounds like a ringing endorsement, until we consider the nature of the statistic more carefully. The Commonwealth Fund's finding is that the NHS is one of the best health systems in the world, based on everything except what happens to the health of the people who use it. It is the equivalent, in sport, of your team doing well on almost every metric – most points scored, number of passes completed, number of meters run, fewest points conceded, best performance ratings. Except, that is, for the fact they come bottom on games won.

Beyond this famous study, a large body of international evidence indicates that the UK health system lags behind.[19] Research from the International Cancer Benchmarking Partnership puts UK cancer outcomes behind comparable health systems. One major paper emerging from the programme and published in *The Lancet* health journal showed that about 5 per cent fewer people survived for five years with breast cancer in the UK than in Sweden; about 10 per cent fewer people survived five years with lung cancer than in Canada; and about 10 per cent fewer people survived ten years with colorectal cancer than in Australia.[20] In sum, before the pandemic, the UK had lower one-year survival rates for stomach, colon, rectal and lung cancer than Australia, Canada, Denmark, Ireland, New Zealand and Norway. A more general study in the *British Medical Journal* showed that the NHS generally performed below average, when looking at as many as 60 different metrics.[21]

International studies on amenable mortality;[22] infant and young person mortality;[23] admission rates of congestive heart failure;[24] and waiting times for knee, cataract and hip replacement all showed similar results.[25]

The political right waste little opportunity in positioning any sign of poor NHS performance in favour of their ideology – and a move to a more explicitly neoliberal or market-based model of healthcare. Covid-19 has provided them with many such opportunities – as per the below from Director of Communications at the Institute for Economic Affairs (IEA), Annabel Denham:

> concerns about the health service's ability to cope with a second wave and a vast backlog of treatments over the course of the winter [strengthen] an already-watertight case for system-level reform of the UK's healthcare system.[26]

The same IEA has since released a full report that linked the leftist nature of the NHS and the country's poor pandemic outcomes.[27] And the IEA are not the only agitators. Among the right's think tanks, the Taxpayers' Alliance can be found making similar arguments.[28] Similar ideas can be found more widely in a range of commentary, opinion pieces, social media feeds, PR work and press releases.[29]

The aggression of these outriders underpins a defensive approach. But, in fact, it's not the only strategy available. The right's critique suggests that the NHS's problems come down to its democratic socialism. But in reality, the NHS never fails because it is too progressive, but rather only ever where it has been artificially constrained by the taint of neoliberalism. The opportunity open to the left is to be honest about the problems our health service faces, to relate them back to questions of political economy, and to use these as a basis to expand our values and advance our health further.

To do this we need to understand where a neoliberal political economy has snuck into our health system, what its consequences have been and then how, through reiteration and modernisation of Bevan's principles, we beat it back.

NEOLIBERAL INFILTRATION

The left's defence has not been enough to prevent the infiltration of the NHS by neoliberal ideas. These haven't come through overt privatisation, but rather through more subtle reforms. Slowly, the NHS has begun to reflect the right's ideology. In turn, that reform has created a chronic fragility – reducing the NHS to an ever more limited safety net and meeting the conditions for the 'buyout'. As such, if 'the defensive' is inevitably about maintaining the status quo, we need to think carefully about what we're defending.

The story of ideological infiltration begins in the 1980s. It was an era of wider political change in Britain: the writings of Friedrich Hayek were ever more in vogue; Ronald Reagan had made his transition from Hollywood to the White House; and Margaret Thatcher had begun what would be one of the most divisive premierships in modern British history. It was during this period that the NHS began a transition from an organisation based on the politics of Nye Bevan and the Labour Party, to one run in line with the principles of Thatcherite neoliberalism.

In 1983, Margaret Thatcher commissioned Sir Roy Griffiths – then chief executive officer of J. Sainsbury's – to review the country's health system. His subsequent report is famous for its contention that:

> If Florence Nightingale were carrying her lamp through the corridors of the NHS today, she would almost certainly be searching for the people in charge.[30]

In answer, he recommended a new model of governance and management. He proposed a shift from 'consensus management' (i.e., management of the NHS by healthcare professionals) to 'general management'. Even more significantly, Griffiths put forward an idea that the NHS engage in competitive tendering, a concept that would lead to a new internal market.

Griffiths imagined a system of competition overseen by professionals with degrees in management theory rather than healthcare or medicine. As one commentator put it in the *Health Service Journal*, it was a transition based on 'business school philosophies and experience from the private sector'.[31] While the NHS would escape Thatcher's wider programme of denationalisation, its governance would begin to embody the logic and teachings of the private sector. Neoliberalism through reform, rather than through sale.

The 'business school' approach to the NHS was formalised in 1989 in the government white paper *Working for Patients*.[32] The document detailed a restructuring of the NHS around competition. Most significantly, two functions of the state – budget holder and service purchaser – were split. Providers became revenue-dependent, and commissioners held the money, forcing the former to compete for financing by the latter.[33] In 1991, a further step was taken, with the expectation imposed on NHS trusts of raising revenue from their patients – ushering in an era of expensive hospital cafes, car parks, vending machines and pay per view TV. Patients were now customers in a system fragmented around the dogma of fierce competition.

NEW LABOUR'S REFORMS

Tony Blair's Labour government offered some initial hope of a quick reversal of the Thatcher reforms. Certainly, that was the promise of the 1997 Labour manifesto.

Early on, momentum seemed to be building towards such a reversal. A new approach to health inequalities formally reallocated money to places that were being poorly served. NHS funding increased substantially. In an early White Paper, the government struck back against the internal market by outlining plans to focus on 'integration'.[34] Blair signalled he was personally on board with the shift, telling an audience at the Lonsdale Medical Centre in 1997 that: 'the White Paper we are publishing today marks a turning point for the NHS. It replaces the internal market with "integrated care". We will put doctors and nurses in the driving seat.'[35]

Hindsight is 20/20 vision, and it all jars with the final legacy. It's now well documented that Tony Blair grew frustrated with his inability to steer change and drive improvement in what he saw as Bevan's 'monolithic', state-led NHS.[36] He became ever more convinced that only fierce competition – that is, a return to and continuation of the Thatcher project – could deliver the change he wanted. The school of public sector management he turned to, which had also formed the basis for Thatcher's reforms, was New Public Management (NPM) – an approach often condensed into the motto: 'targets and markets'. It was this adage that, in the end, would really define Blair's health vision.

In came the National Service Frameworks – imposing ambitious, comprehensive, long-term and very top-down targets. 'Strategic Health Authorities' were created to oversee delivery by individual providers, with the power to withhold funding when the centre's expectations weren't met. Fundholding was reinvigorated, alongside strict financial budgeting. Competition was reiterated, with new restraints on collaboration – to the point that providers could not help each other out with small loans. Independent Providers were given a stronger foothold, to compete with and drive on the public sector. A new Quality Outcomes Framework constituted a financial lever to drive up the quantity of specific activities. From 1999 onwards, the new Health Secretary Alan Milburn took on a mission to reallocate significant power to the patient: a choose and book service, review systems and a new look NHS website branded 'NHS Choices' all followed.

The logic was simple. Blair concluded that Thatcher's restructuring of the NHS for competition could be combined with ever more extensive targets, linked directly to funding (a public sector equivalent to profit). Trusts could be made further accountable to budgets and revenue (a public sector equivalent to the profit motive). Greater fragmentation would induce greater competition. And stronger patient choice would create winners and losers, and drive competition (a public sector equivalent to supply and demand). It is entirely in line with the 'business school' ideas introduced by Griffiths – and one New Labour were convinced could herald a new era of infinite improvement.

Undeniably, the quality of healthcare provision improved across some significant metrics during Blair's three terms. However, given that he increased NHS funding massively, after several years of stagnation, this is difficult to attribute directly to his theories of reform rather than to the extra money.[37]

In fact, there are reasons to think that these reforms constrained the NHS's potential, rather than releasing it. Moreover, reports from 2007 remind us that Blair did not leave office with a clearly positive legacy. NHS managers were left dissatisfied by the sheer number of targets enforced upon them, with some suggesting they were wrestling with as many as 300 centrally imposed standards. Big ambitions on health inequalities had translated into a nearly negligible impact, and regular stories about postcode lotteries – rife variations in access to care and treatments based on where one happened to live – continued to dominate the media. The stated prioritisation of patient choice seemed to clash with rising public dissatisfaction with how the health service was run. Despite the money invested, healthcare providers faced major debts and deficits in 2007. And the system continued to struggle with the severe fragmentation and problems with collaboration associated with competition policies.[38]

In other cases, there were scandals within the NHS that suggested the private sector's logic had been implemented far too uncritically. In the private sector, it is well established that the pressures of continuous growth and the profit motive can lead to underhand, undesirable, or exploitative practices – to the detriment of both workers and consumers. In the 2000s, there were echoes of this in the NHS. For example, in 2007, Julie Bailey's mother died in Stafford Hospital. The death opened scrutiny on an unjustifiably high mortality rate among patients being treated there, particularly emergency cases. The Francis Inquiry, convened to investigate the hospital, would find hundreds of unnecessary deaths at the hands of systematic neglect – implicating a toxic culture, unsafe staffing, pace-setting techniques and institutional bullying. In short, the pressures of competition as dictated by NPM.[39]

CAMERON'S COALITION GOVERNMENT

Margaret Thatcher had put in place the structures for NPM whilst Tony Blair put in place the tools to operationalise it. David Cameron took a next, critical step.

In many ways, the coalition's brand of austerity was entirely consistent with the principles of NPM – only now, 'with less' was the keystone. That is, the tools of NPM introduced over three decades were relentlessly adapted to drive efficiency savings, control cost and reduce capacity. As Cameron himself phrased it in a 2012 speech to factory workers in Basildon: 'what you call austerity, I call efficiency'.[40]

An early example was the 'Nicholson challenge' – implemented early in the Coalition years.[41] Under the 'challenge', the NHS was charged with finding £20 billion in efficiency savings by 2015. It would commence a trend – with the NHS's Five Year Forward View strategy asking for similar 'efficiency' savings. Today, it is still common to hear the frustration of senior health officials and civil servants as they find their proposals for highly necessary investment accepted by HM Treasury – provided they can be funded through productivity savings, rather than by actual money.

In the end, David Cameron delivered on his manifesto pledge not to cut funding for the NHS. However, the austerity decade oversaw the biggest deceleration in health spending in history. As the Institute for Fiscal Studies have shown, NHS spending grew at an average annual rate of 3.5 per cent between formation and 1979. It grew at 3.3 per cent per year under the Thatcher and Major governments, between 1978/9 and 1996/7. The Blair and Brown governments also oversaw significant health expansion – of 6 per cent per year on average (though they also arguably proved money alone is not enough without strategy). But the rate of spending decreased in the Coalition years to just 1.0 per cent – followed by 1.6 per cent between 2014/15 and 2018/19.[42]

On paper, it doesn't constitute a cut to NHS funding – but rather a subjection of the NHS to the brutal reality of rising population health need and national demand. The rises in funding – particularly during the coalition years – only just outstripped England's population growth of 0.8 per cent. But once all the variables that increase demand on the health service are considered – an aging population, growing population health needs, the requirements of new technologies and treatments, changes in NHS pay – the funding needed just to maintain the NHS comes to 3.3 per cent. That means the coalition and Conservative governments in the 2010s oversaw major and sustained funding cuts in the NHS.

This subjugation of the NHS to demand pressures is a strategy designed to force a system-wide search for all possible efficiencies, for any 'spare' capacity that can be cut, for any spending commitment or pay rise that can be resisted. While Covid means NHS funding rises now look far more respectable than ten years ago, the same strategy can still be observed at work. In September 2021, the Prime Minister and Chancellor of the Exchequer introduced a new Health and Social Care Levy, funded by a rise to National Insurance Contributions. The money raised meant around £15 billion more funding for the NHS over three years than previously planned. But just days before, extensive research jointly undertaken by the NHS' own representative bodies – NHS Confederation and NHS Providers – had put the direct costs of Covid-19 at £10 billion per year, double what had been allocated.[43] It is another example, even in the pandemic, of the NHS being forced to find efficiencies, just to get by. It is a regime entirely consistent with the treatment of the health service under austerity, and one that both suppresses performance in the short-term and undermines resilience to shocks in the long-term.

CHRONIC FRAGILITY AND COVID-19

Covid-19 provides a case study in the consequences of several decades of neoliberal infiltration. It demonstrates how the shift to a NPM model based on 'targets and markets' and 'do more with less' created a chronic fragility that transformed the NHS from Bevan's comprehensive service to a more limited safety net.

The Partnership for Health System Sustainability and Resilience[44] – a global partnership evaluating resilience across different national health systems – has set out a comprehensive set of measures that define the ability of health services to 'continually deliver their key functions' (including during crisis events). These cover:

- The number and location of beds
- The number and organisation of the workforce
- Deployment of innovation – whether in the organisation of the system, available technology, use of digital and AI tools, or the provision of the best treatments for all those who need them
- A comprehensive health budget (both capital and resource)

These metrics are an excellent starting point from which to explore how, in all but name, reform has undermined the NHS's universality.

Beds were an immediate focus when Covid-19 hit in Winter 2020. Two types of hospital bed are particularly important in reacting to a disease like Covid-19: critical care beds, where the sickest patients are cared for, and general hospital beds, which are more common. As a country, we had too few of both.

In January 2020, the month that would become the quiet before the storm, just 700 critical care beds were open and available in England.[45] These were not equally distributed over the country either. The NHS commissioning region with the fewest beds was the South West. For those reading this book from cities like Exeter, Bristol, or Plymouth, you may be frightened to learn that just 51 critical beds were available for the whole of your region when the pandemic began.[46]

Acute beds were also in short supply. Since 2010, about 10,000 hospital beds have been closed in England. In turn, the UK entered Covid with just 2.5 hospital beds available for every 1,000 people, whereas Germany had 8 and South Korea had 12.[47]

But there is a more important metric than total stock when it comes to beds: occupancy rate. It is possible to have a small number of beds, and still provide safe care – for example, if community care infrastructure is extensive. The best evidence is that safe hospitals have at least 15 per cent of their beds free, to ensure that they can deal with demand spikes.[48] It is a level of occupancy we have not been able to maintain, on aggregate, for years.[49] Just before the outbreak, more than four out of five hospitals had occupancy levels above that safe 85 per cent level. Three out of five had occupancies over 90 per cent. And a full one in four had occupancies over 95 per cent. This would have left them with too little capacity to manage demand, and so no choice but to retract universal care, in the face of even a much smaller health shock.[50]

Of course, hospital beds are next to useless without a team of healthcare professionals to staff them. And when the Covid-19 outbreak began, the UK was in the grips of the NHS's worst ever capacity crisis – driven by the fact we have one of the smallest healthcare workforces in the world, given the size of our population. For every 1,000 people living here, we have just eight nurses and three doctors – both below the average in the OECD.[51] For every 100 people over 65, we have just three professionals providing 'long-term care' – compared to 13 in Norway and an OECD average of five.[52] If the UK – a population with relatively high health needs – were to recruit enough workers to break into the top quarter of OECD nations, we would need hundreds of thousands more nurses and tens of thousands more doctors.[53] These are skilled professionals, who take years to train – meaning gaps cannot easily be filled when a crisis strikes. When it comes to workforce, there isn't really an equivalent to opening a field hospital.

The resources those workers then have at their disposal are also comparably poor. Compared to international standards, the UK offers less of the best treatments to patients. Every year, the government compares the UK's uptake of the best medicines with that of other European countries. In 2019, just 20 per cent of the new medicines available elsewhere were available here, despite having been formally approved based on cost effectiveness, safety and efficacy. It is the same story when it comes to health technology. Compared to other countries, the UK has fewer CT scanners and MRI machines – fundamental pieces of technology for diagnostics. In the OECD, the average is 17 MRI machines and 25 CT scanners per million people. The UK had fewer than 10 per million.

It is the fragility implicit in the dogmatic implementation of 'do more with less' in our NHS that Covid-19 has exposed.

CHRONIC FRAGILITY BEFORE COVID

There's an obvious defence here: namely, that Covid was an unprecedented crisis. Yet, in fact, it wasn't just during the pandemic that fragility was evident. As much as it undermined resilience to crisis, it was undermining people's healthcare before the virus struck.

In 2018, a report by the NHS Confederation established the idea of the 'all year-round crisis' in the NHS.[54] The report systematically demonstrated how a growing mismatch between NHS capacity (supply) and national need (demand) was making it ever more difficult for the system to guarantee people timely, personalised, effective care.

In A&E, they showed a 7.3 per cent increase in attendances between Summer 2013/14 and Summer 2017/18. Over the same period, outpatient attendance at general or acute services increased by 10.6 per cent. The number of people with learning disabilities, autism or adult mental health needs had increased 10 per cent between 2015/16 and 2016/17. Evidence pointed to community services 'running at full capacity'. The number of 999 calls increased by 21 per cent. Yet, across these settings, capacity had either decreased or remained stagnant.

The reality is, without disputing the fact the pandemic has caused clear disruption in the health service, lots of problems we face today are entirely in line with pre-pandemic trends. Take cancer. Data from the Global Burden of Disease datasets show years of improvement in both the death rate and the rate of Disability Adjusted Life Years lost to cancer. Then, from around 2012, the progress begins to tail off. By the end of the decade, it is in full reverse. Had the improvements observed between 1990 and 2010 continued through the last decade, 15,000 fewer people would have died from the four most common cancers (lung, prostate, breast and colorectal). And there would have been 300,000 fewer Disability Adjusted Life Years lost to the same conditions.[55] The British Heart Foundation have identified the same trends in heart disease, with Covid disruptions continuing and accentuating a downward trajectory – rather than creating it.[56]

Evidently, Covid-19 has done severe damage, accentuated by our lack of resilience coming into the pandemic. But we must be careful that the exceptional circumstances of a pandemic do not obscure the structural, political, and ideological underpinnings of our current crisis. It is tempting – emerging on both the right and the left – to explain all instances of NHS strain and poor access to health services through the prism of the pandemic. But in many cases, the blame lies with the failed policies of neoliberalism and austerity.

PUT 'UNIVERSALISING THE BEST' BACK IN OUR NHS

A defensive strategy makes it very difficult to think of ways to expand the NHS and its universality, as opposed to focusing on (at best) simply maintaining it. This is reflected in the policy ideas that have gained momentum – including Renationalisation[57] or an NHS Reinstatement Bill[58] – which are too limited or backward looking to found the distinctly left-wing, forward looking vision of the NHS that re-expressing its universality requires.

If what we need is a re-expression of universality, there is no better anchor than Bevan's principle of 'Universalise the Best' (UTB). Importantly, this is not about a nostalgia-led argument for a return to the NHS's 1948 form – when it was organised around meeting acute health conditions, and its budget was just over £437 million (compared to c.£150 billion today). Rather, it is about expanding and modernising NHS universality – by bringing its reach into new spaces, making it resilient to rising demand and ridding it of institutional injustices that exclude vulnerable people. The five shifts we can coalesce around are outlined below and summarised in *Table 1.1*

Table 1.1   Five Shifts to Universalise the Best in the NHS

	New Public Management	Universalising the Best
Extent of Universality	Minimum feasible	Maximum possible
Capacity for Universality	Skeleton-crew	Oversupply
Resilience of Universality	Resilience considered inefficient	Resilience considered essential
Approach to Health	NHS as a treatment service	NHS as a wellness service
Access to Universality	Exclusionary	Inclusive

EXTEND UNIVERSALITY

In tandem with cost-constraint, a culture of risk-aversion embedded by the NPM paradigm is key to explaining the discrepancy between provision of the best tools and medicines to all in the UK – and in other health systems.

Risk aversion is clear in the performance metrics it prioritises and the targets it sets: patient safety, waiting times and financial sustainability. These targets are, in and of themselves, not necessarily bad things

– safety, particularly, is obviously important. But they are targets exclusively focused on managing risk, and therefore managing costs, rather than on alternatives like quality improvement.

This dominance of risk management has very real consequences. Analysis has shown that if the UK were able to meet the standards of health set by its international peers in just four areas – stroke, cancer, cardiovascular disease and dementia – it would add £20 billion to the economy per year; save £10 billion for the NHS per year; and, most importantly, save 20,000 lives per year.[59]

There are many studies and reports that ask why the NHS often struggles, more than other healthcare systems, to get the best technology, medicines, tools and care to all its patients. It is a strange state of affairs, given distribution of the best healthcare was such a clear goal behind the NHS's initial creation. Many of these explorations end up displaying a sense of fatalism in their conclusions: they argue the NHS is just too complicated to ever get a grip on scaling or spreading good practices or lacks the appetite for innovation found in the private sector. The experience of Covid-19 makes these conclusions appear highly suspect.

During the pandemic, something changed: things that we'd been talking about spreading across the health service were scaled, often very quickly. Take general practice. There has long been an ambition to move towards digitally enabled general practice. In 2019, 71 per cent of general practice consultations happened face to face. As of April 2020, 71 per cent of consultation took place digitally.[60] While there are still questions to answer, and urgent questions in the case of the impact of digital exclusions, it still stands up as a remarkable pace of change. Before 2020, many would have thought it impossible.

A digital shift in primary care is not the only such instance. Clinicians have identified a whole host of examples that they find valuable, including rapid access to intermediate care and community assessment, joint working protocols with care homes and 'virtual wards' creating hospitals at home.[61] These are evidenced, have been possible for a long time and are demonstrative of how the NHS has been artificially held back from delivering the frontier of what is possible.

I wanted to understand how this happened so quickly during Covid, when such changes had seemed so difficult before. So, in Summer 2020 I interviewed some GPs as part of a wider exploration of how things changed during the pandemic. Across the board, they affirmed three things:

1. The NHS had developed a very clear sense of mission (fight the virus).
2. The government had got rid of all the bureaucracy and hoops that clinicians had previously been asked to jump through before changing how things are done in their practice.
3. They could access a little money to help get things done, whereas before even small budget requests involved strenuous business cases and were likely to be denied.

More specifically, they talked about how all the artificial instruments used to manage risk and money in a system run according to NPM – like onerous business cases, the policing of collaboration, the abolition of clinical networks and consensus decision making, the tight controls on even small amounts of money – had, at least temporarily, disappeared.

This opens an opportunity for a radical change in culture. At the moment, the health service is organised to react – often discordantly – to instances where patient safety is put at risk, or money unnecessarily wasted. But a missed opportunity to use a new tool, prescribe a new medicine, or try a better practice still causes avoidable harm, disease, or death. Put simply, missed opportunities can have the same human cost as safety incidents. Moreover, being better at taking these opportunities and spreading them does not require us to accept undue risk. Rather, it relies on significantly improving how patients and professionals talk about risk, when making shared decisions on care and treatment.

That is, it requires us to be perennially unsatisfied with the NHS remaining in stasis, against a backdrop of stunning scientific advances and rapidly growing population health need.

INCREASE CAPACITY

Universality relies on resources. And in the NHS, the resource that is most precious isn't, surprisingly, money. It's workers. UTB relies on our ability to end a boom and bust cycle that has plagued our health workforce, and our ability to sustain the most ambitious definitions of universality.

'Boom and bust' conjures up an image of sleepless nights for economists, but is equally salient in the NHS. It refers to our predilection for huge workforce shortages. A historical perspective shows the workforce crisis of the 1940s, when the NHS was formed, and needed an immediate uplift in staff. There was another major crisis in the 1960s, when Enoch Powell (of all people) led a globe-trotting international recruitment campaign targeted at international doctors.[62] There was a further crisis in the 1990s and early 2000s, particularly in the nursing profession.[63] And then there was the pre-Covid crisis when shortages and vacancies blighted nearly every category of health profession.[64] If we include Covid as another, distinct crisis, that's five major busts in just over 70 years.

We run into this problem because, consistent with my discussion of NPM, we have an NHS obsessed with 'just enough'. In workforce planning, this translates to the health sector's own version of 'just in time' delivery. The idea of ever producing *more* doctors, nurses, or other healthcare professionals than the NHS needs is intolerable to the political and policy decision makers across the country. They find the idea of a vacancy far more palatable than the idea of investing in the training of a UK health professional who plies their trade outside the NHS or, worse, outside the country.

There is a relatively simple solution – a shift, in the post-pandemic era, to a policy of oversupply. Simply put, that would rest on an independent body estimating the amount and type of healthcare workers we'll need in the future, and the country then training more professionals than the scenario demands.

In some ways, this will be more acceptable in the twenty-first century than it ever was in the twentieth. As compared to the past 100 years, much of the world faces a shortfall in its health and care workforce – as their population increases, their middle classes grow and the average age of their population rises. There is now a global and humanitarian case, as well as a domestic one, for training more healthcare professionals than the NHS needs.

This will mean some very technical discussions about training places, education pathways and workforce composition. But my research has focused on a second, equally important question: how can the NHS be an employer that actually attracts and retains workers?

There is a very clear discrepancy between people's love for the NHS as a care provider, and what people think about the NHS as an employer. Almost eight in ten people think the NHS is crucial to British society and must be maintained. But only half of the same group would recommend a friend or family member consider a career in the NHS.[65]

One of the best places to start is the most obvious – pay. The suppression of pay in the NHS has been a direct and intentional consequence of a decade of hostile government policy. Most notable was the government public sector pay freeze, beginning in 2010. The result of this decision was a large real term pay cut. At the time of writing,[66] my analysis indicates that the average nurse or midwife has lost around 10 per cent of their pay, compared to a decade ago, after accounting for inflation.[67]

Cuts to pay come with very real consequences. Research carried out during the Winter 2020/1 peak of the Covid-19 pandemic showed that 30 per cent of nurses were relying on borrowed money to pay for essentials. Four in ten had skipped meals to feed their families. Two in three were working overtime to pay their bills. Use of food banks was growing ever more common.[68]

Pay justice is important, for recruitment and retention, but it shouldn't be the sum of our ambition. My research with healthcare workers has consistently shown other needs – including housing, childcare provision, flexible working, progression and time for rest. The hours that healthcare professionals work make it very difficult to balance childcare commitments, particularly if working fulltime, or if sharing childcare with a partner also in the health sector. Rising housing costs put secure, affordable accommodation out of the hands of many in the NHS – represented, anecdotally but shockingly, by NHS workers receiving eviction notices at the beginning of the Covid-19 pandemic by landlords who didn't want to run the risk of key workers living in their buildings. Equally indicative of housing insecurity is 2019 research by the New Economics Foundation, which found that two in three homes built on surplus NHS land between 2017 and 2018 would be unaffordable to a nurse on an average salary, and that just 1 in 20 would qualify as genuinely affordable socially rented housing.[69]

What all this indicates is a relatively simple point. People who work for the NHS want their employment to offer them security, fulfilment of their basic needs, flexibility and hope. They want it to be a place they have the chance to reach their career aspirations, where they can balance work with life and where they can benefit from the security of decent pay, a decent home and decent breaks from the workplace. Until the public sector offers workers those basics, it will struggle to attract enough people into roles, and it will struggle to retain the people it does have through their career.

Perhaps most urgent is action on mental health. In 2021, I ran a survey alongside my colleague Dr Parth Patel, to understand the state of burnout after the second Covid-19 peak. The research showed that 65 per cent of workers were physically exhausted, 70 per cent were mentally exhausted, 50 per cent were working understaffed shifts at least once a week, 25 per cent were turning to alcohol or drugs weekly to cope with work-stress and 5 per cent – equivalent to 80,000 workers – were having suicidal thoughts. The workers had a very clear sense of where the blame lay. Nine in ten said it was down to delayed government policy during the pandemic and a late lockdown. Eight in ten said it was because the NHS had been run so hot during austerity. And seven in ten put it down to the country's unacceptable levels of health and social inequality.[70]

Sadly, this is another instance of Covid-19 exposing a trend that already existed. The health and care workforce aren't in crisis just because of a dreadful two years fighting Covid. They are in crisis because that awful 24 months came on the back of a dreadful decade for workers. According to the NHS's official staff survey, the number of workers experiencing illness due to work-related stress had reached 500,000 in 2019 and nearly 600,000 in 2020.[71] It translates into severe mental health consequences. Mind say four in ten GPs experience mental illness.[72] A paper by Dame Clare Gerada, in the *British Journal of General Practice*, demonstrated how medical professionals experience much higher rates of suicide than the wider population[73] – with female doctors at 2.5 to 4 times the risk of other professionals by some estimates.[74] We cannot expect the best care, from a sustainable number of workers, while we ask that NHS workers simply accept severe mental illness as an occupational hazard.

In sum, our workforce undersupply model is built on a vicious cycle. The life the NHS offers its workers isn't good enough to attract enough new people into its various professions. In turn, shortages drive burnout and poor mental health. More people are put off joining, or otherwise leave the sector. And all the while, the Treasury justifies its chronic underinvestment in workers with the phrase 'labour market conditions' – based on the misguided short-termism that wider economic malaise provides an excuse to suppress pay, terms, conditions and wellbeing in the health service, rather than an obligation to lift it up.

EMBED RESILIENCE

Expanding universality means maintaining the capacity to provide everyone with the best care, even during health shocks. A combination of an ageing population and – as Chapter 5 will discuss – global health vulnerability mean we need to be prepared to handle spikes in demand.

It has not always been the case that the NHS was so susceptible to demand shocks. It has been driven and normalised by a ruthless focus on efficiency, over any concept of resilience or sustainability. The kind of extra capacity that protects us when things go wrong has been redefined, in the last four decades, as needless waste.

I have come across some astounding cases of efficiency being justified over resilience, even in the face of evidence. For some, their reaction to the evidence in this chapter is to acknowledge that there are gaps in provision, but to argue that the country at least delivers said healthcare services at a very, very good price. That is, there is a relatively dominant line of argument that sees the data I've outlined here as a success of efficiency and value, rather than a failure of quality and resilience. That's a big problem, and a narrative that must be challenged and changed.

One of the key learnings of Covid-19 will be that this efficiency paradigm doesn't even work on its own terms. Rather, in its short-termism, it represents an approach that inevitably costs more money when all is said and done. This is plain from a macro-perspective. When a disease that preyed on underlying health conditions and health inequality hit, this country had large numbers of people living with avoidable health conditions and severe levels of health inequality. This made the economic consequences of Covid-19 deeper, and demanded more invasive, regressive public health interventions to stem the damage of the virus. Small investments in health in the decades before Covid-19 would have had huge value propositions and return on investment in pre-empting such a health crisis.

There are some tangible case studies, too – perhaps the best of which is the cost of the Nightingale hospitals. The Nightingale fleet was only necessary because of a lack of capacity in the health service. They were required to maintain confidence in the NHS avoiding collapse, because bed numbers, occupancy levels and ICU capacity were all uncertain in Spring 2020. No data embodies this fact better than the fact the Nightingales were hardly used. The London site saw just 54 patients during the pandemic's first wave. Estimates suggest that spending on the Nightingale's will total somewhere between £500 million and £1 billion. Some estimates put the cost at over £1 million per patient in the year 2020, a cost equal to fifty cancer treatments.

Had we embedded a UTB principle before the pandemic, we would have secured the same surge capacity far more proactively. For example, evidence has pointed out a dual problem with hospital discharge in the NHS – namely, some patients being discharged far too quickly (and therefore returning) and others far too late. The combined cost of these two trends is an estimated £3 billion per year.[75] Investing the Nightingale funding into better discharge processes and more community access before the pandemic – rather than waiting until a crisis hit – could have freed up hospital beds, saved money and tangibly helped people. It could, indicatively, have funded a massive rise in community capacity: 50 million hours of community care to support discharge, 20–30 million physiotherapy services or 17 million one-to-one occupation therapy sessions. All of these are excellent ways of improving discharge.

The challenge is finding a simple policy lever through which to embed maintenance resilience as the new common sense in health service management. Any solution will need to ensure straying from resilience costs political capital. In 2020, I proposed one such approach.[76] I suggested that the UK government borrow from economic policy's 'fiscal rules' and introduce 'health and care resilience rules'. In the Treasury, the fiscal rules are designed to embed political accountability around consistent and long-term focused economic policy. In health, these rules could include:

1. *A Capacity Rule*: We should open enough hospital beds to reach safe occupancy levels in hospital.[77] Thereafter, any hospital bed closures should only be allowed if there is pre-emptive and equal investment in other settings (home care, community care, social care).
2. *A Staffing Rule*: A commitment to reach and maintain, at the very least, the average workforce per capita in comparator countries – across medical, nursing, allied health, ambulance and community professions.
3. *A Modernisation Rule*: A commitment to making available at least the same number of National Institute for Health and Care Excellence (NICE) approved and cost effective treatments to England patients as made available in other advanced countries – and to ensure we match other countries on technology, data and digital tools.
4. *A Sustainable Funding Rule*: NHS funding made equal, in the first instance, to the average investment in the G7 (ignoring one-off Covid-19 investments) – with funding used to enable transformation and resilience.

Combined with regular reporting, these rules could help set expectations and ensure political cost when those expectations are breached.

FROM TREATMENT TO WELLNESS

The trajectory of changing population health needs means NHS universality will only be assured when it can provide for the reality of multiple conditions and wide inequalities.

The reality of people being diagnosed with multiple chronic conditions – perhaps arthritis, combined with depression or anxiety, alongside COPD or angina – means changing our model to one that can provide more holistic support. People no longer need just intensive support in hospitals (a treatment service). They need help to cope with chronic conditions, and to still live brilliant lives within their homes and community (a wellness service).

There are emerging examples of services yielding fantastic results by going *to* people in the places they live, making better use of community and charity services,[78] and treating the whole person, not just their illness.

In Glasgow, a programme called 'Improving the Cancer Journey' was launched in 2014. It serves a community support service, providing everyone with an individualised assessment and care to local people diagnosed with cancer. The needs assessment covers not just physical, but emotional, family, practical and spiritual needs – going far beyond ideas and services traditionally seen as within the health service's remit. Its focus on outreach and presence in the place where people actually live – rather than in out of the way, medicalised settings – meant it was incredibly beneficial and accessible for people living in more deprived parts of the city, and those living with more complicated or multiple physical and mental health needs.[79] Elsewhere, 'hub models' – community clinics with GPs, but also local authority, charity, co-operative and voluntary sector services – are having an impressive impact.

The problem is, these kinds of services are currently only possible in isolated instances, and where they have access to voluntary sector funding. They do not represent fundamental changes in the NHS's publicly funded service offer.

Indeed, estimates suggest community care services and infrastructure have actually been significantly cut back in recent years.[80] Changing this trajectory, and extending the NHS beyond hospitals, is critical to Universalising the Best, ensuring equality of access to health services and ensuring universality in the face of changing health challenges in the decades to come.

ELIMINATE INSTITUTIONAL INJUSTICE

An obvious case of institutional injustice in the NHS is the interaction between British colonialism and the origins and evolution of the National Health Service. The NHS's existence was only made possible by the international workforce that staffed it, upon its creation in 1948. Indeed, its existence came in the same year that the passengers of the HMT Empire Windrush landed in the Port of Tilbury. They landed to find a newly formed NHS in desperate need of their labour,[81] and many would go on to staff this ambitious new public service.[82]

Ever since, our NHS has remained viable because of its global workforce. Throughout history, we have answered workforce shortages with massive international recruitment campaigns. Before he spoke of 'Rivers of Blood', Enoch Powell launched and led an overseas campaign to find and recruit trained doctors – bringing in 18,000 new staff from India and Pakistan alone.[83] Today, the UK workforce is more international than almost any other in the world. 15.4 per cent of UK nurses and 29.2 per cent of UK physicians were trained in another country – compared to an average amongst EU 15 countries of 4.2 and 15.1 per cent respectively.[84]

This is often presented as a point of pride. Matt Hancock MP has talked about 'the benefits of a diverse, international workforce' and about 'welcoming even more incredible talent to our health system'.[85] At his 2018 conference speech, the Labour Shadow Minister for Health Jonathan Ashworth gave his thanks to 'those who have come from across the world to care for our sick and elderly whether from the EU, the Indian sub-continent and yes the Windrush generation too'.[86]

By ignoring that this system is built on the back of exploitation, such uncritical pride amounts to rank hypocrisy. Despite its reliance on healthcare professionals trained in Britain's former colonies, the NHS was an integral participant in the formation of the 'hostile environment' pioneered by Theresa May as Home Secretary. For example, new regulations introduced in 2015 require NHS Trusts to charge people who are not eligible for NHS care at 150 per cent of the cost of that care. The same regulations introduced an Immigration Health Surcharge – a fee levied on UK VISA applications, including for NHS workers, on top of other Home Office immigration charges.[87]

The scheme serves a dual purpose within government policy. First, it allows the government to further embed their culture of 'do more with less'. Even though the government's own estimates put the cost of NHS 'misuse' by international visitors at just £300 million, an extensive effort to reclaim these funds communicates the extent to which they'll go to retain money. More importantly, as highlighted by grassroot campaign group Docs not Cops, it helps create an environment of surveillance and overt repression. That is, a legal duty on NHS Trusts to charge is also a legal duty on NHS Trusts to undertake extensive immigration checks, and to employ their privileged access to data in support of the hostile environment. It is even more powerful because it comes through a service that we cannot do without.[88]

Put simply: the NHS only functions because of the contributions of an international workforce – past and present. In many cases, their education and training has been funded abroad, and the extent to which the UK relies on international recruitment often draws workers away from countries where they are also needed. The World Health Organisation estimates that 18 million more health workers are needed to achieve universal healthcare in low and lower-middle income countries by 2030 – a target from which the UK evidently detracts.[89] And yet, those same workers have been deployed as part of a regime designed to police migrants, control borders and enact a hostile environment.

The severe health impacts of the Windrush scandal – whereby hundreds of Commonwealth citizens, many from the 'Windrush' generation, were wrongly deported or denied legal rights – brought this story full circle. The policing of access to the NHS constituted a denial of healthcare for many who had come to the UK as part of the same Windrush generation that filled the NHS immediate labour needs in the 1940s. Of course, the right to healthcare should be a human right for all migrants – regardless of their economic contribution. Nonetheless, juxtaposing the economic contribution demanded of migrant people by the British state, with its reluctance to extend human rights and the welfare state, gives a clear sign of our hypocrisy and of health's continued struggles with colonialism and colonial structures.

Institutional injustice in health is not just about individual scandals. If the NHS is a system tainted by colonialism, then the impact can be seen in how well its services are designed around the needs of people from

Black, Asian, or Minority Ethnic backgrounds. From this perspective, we see a system that translates colonialism into a universally poorer offer for many people today.

Where there is data – and health data on ethnicity is often limited – there are signs of a big problem in how Black patients are treated within the NHS. For example, every year, the NHS releases results of its Cancer Patient Experience Survey – giving a comprehensive overview of what people think about their cancer care. There are sixty questions, all covering different interactions with the health service. Nine of those questions do not have a breakdown for ethnicity. Of the remaining fifty-one questions, my analysis for this book shows that Black people have worse experiences on 40 metrics. People from Asian backgrounds have worse experiences on 46 metrics. Particularly notable disparities include:

- Black and Asian people having to visit their GP more times before they are referred, indicating their symptoms are not taken as seriously
- Black and Asian people more often indicating their test results were not explained in a way they could understand
- Black and Asian people more likely to indicate they were not treated with respect and dignity in hospitals

These are indicative of an NHS that remains structured in a way that is discriminatory, more amenable to the needs of white people and retains the fingerprints of institutionalised, enduring colonialism.[90]

To some extent, this is depressingly unsurprising, given who designs and leads the NHS as a health institute (and has done through its whole history). Despite the introduction of a Workforce Race Equality Standard (WRES) in 2015, problems continue in Black representation, particularly in leadership positions. Across the whole country, 20 per cent of staff in NHS Trusts and Clinical Commissioning Groups are from a Black, Asian or minority ethnic (BME) background. But they represent just 8 per cent of NHS board members.[91] And they are significantly underrepresented in the highest pay bands – with just 6.5 per cent of BME workers in 'very senior management' positions.[92]

This isn't down to a deficit in talent, and there are signs that people from minority ethnic groups have their progress stymied by bosses and colleagues. Research from just last year found that workers from minority ethnic backgrounds were twice as likely to have experienced discrimination or unfair treatment from a colleague or a manager.[93]

Unsurprisingly, a system designed by white British people and managed by white British people provides better access and outcomes for white British people. Recent government research has shown that Black women are both the most likely to develop depression and anxiety disorders, and the least likely to receive mental health treatment for these same disorders.[94] Worse, Black adults are significantly more likely to be sectioned under the Mental Health Act.[95] There are discrepancies outside of mental health, too. For instance, the end-of-life care charity Marie Curie found discrepancies in whether someone has dignified, high quality palliative care – attributable to race – meaning people dying less dignified and more painful deaths on for no clinically justifiable reason.[96]

This kind of exclusion is in line with the priorities of the system that has developed over the last four decades. A focus on financial sustainability, one-size-fits-all targets, competition and efficiency actively incentivises healthcare providers to ignore those with more complicated (and expensive) health needs. That is, it encourages them to sustain existing inequality. A left approach based on romanticising the NHS is, equally, poorly optimised to challenge this reality. In approaching health as an agenda we've won – and a status quo to preserve – we lack the natural scepticism of state institutions found in activism against prisons, the police or the Home Office's deportation regime.

Of course, it's important not to erase areas where this problem is focused on by excellent grassroots movements. Decolonising Contraception, MedAct and Black Lives Matter have all done excellent work in pushing these important issues and stories into prominence. A definitive test of our movement will be whether these kinds of experiences and statistics can come to drive the same campaign activity seen around questions of privatisation; or when deaths from poor health attributable to racism cause the same outcry as deaths attributable to racism within the Metropolitan Police.

We need to be able to look honestly at the problems within our NHS, bring that radical critique back to questions of politics and ideology, and push transformative justice. It is a need that conflicts with the desire to defend and romanticise the NHS. It is one of the clearest reasons for an adjustment in our movement's strategy.

2
The Social Justice Frontier

Our ambition cannot end with the National Health Service, no matter how much more expansive. Health improvement and health justice, the twin aims of this book, demand we focus beyond just one institution and look at public health as a whole system.

Just as an economist might be interested in both the total sum of wealth, and how that is then shared out, the coming chapters are interested both in how we can increase our stock of good health and, perhaps more importantly, how we can create a public health system that distributes good health fairly.

This line of enquiry brings us back to Orwell's observation, with which I opened the book: why is that some conditions seem to only (or more aggressively or more regularly) attack people at the lower income levels?

Orwell immediately turns to hospitals and health settings for his own explanation in *How the Poor Die*, a premonition perhaps of contemporary NHS-centrism. But there is another work from the progressive canon that provides an even more accurate explanation of the political economy of public health today.

WHY WAS TINY TIM SICK?

Charles Dickens' *A Christmas Carol* follows the archetypal miser Ebenezer Scrooge, a man who is mean with his money, even to his own detriment, who neither invests in his own comforts, nor entertains philanthropy. Bob Cratchit is the unlucky clerk in Scrooge's employ, and as a result faces a severe combination of low pay, long hours and poor living conditions. His poverty is compounded by circumstance. Bob and wife Emily have four children – the youngest of which, Tiny Tim, is seriously ill. Dickens describes the boy as cheerful and full of spirit, as per his famous line: 'God bless us, everyone'. But his illness is worse than can be solved by a positive disposition. When Scrooge is visited by the Ghost of Christmas Yet to Come, he sees that, should the timeline continue unchanged, Tiny Tim will die.

Dickens does not give Tiny Tim a diagnosis, but many have since taken on the medical detective work. A review by Dr Russell Chesney in *the Archives of Paediatric and Adolescent Medicine* summarises the most likely suggestions: Rickets; Tuberculosis (or a combination of the two); Renal Tubular Acidosis (Type 1);[1] or simple malnutrition.[2] These hypotheses help us understand what Tiny Tim would have needed to survive.

A common thread among all these potential diagnoses is that he would have needed interventions that sit outside the gift of even the modern NHS. Malnutrition is a disease of diet, rickets either of diet or exposure to sunlight. Renal Tubular Acidosis would have demanded exercise, sunlight, better diet, or even a supplement of sodium bicarbonate. Chronic tuberculosis could be prevented, or managed, with increased Vitamin D[3] – particularly, if diagnosed in tandem with rickets.[4]

As the Ghost of Christmas Present shows Ebenezer Scrooge, Tiny Tim's ailment would have been fatal should his poverty have continued. His salvation is not down to a new medical discovery, the creation of a new health service, a lucky improvement in condition, or advancement through individual merit on the part of his father. Rather, the difference between Tiny Tim dying and surviving is the reformation of Ebenezer Scrooge – and the fairer living standards that become available to the whole Cratchit family thereafter. That is, the end of his family's poverty saves his life.

THE TWENTY-FIRST CENTURY TINY TIMS

Two centuries on, *A Christmas Carol* is remarkably in-line with the workings of health distribution and injustice in Britain today. The link between poor health and poverty has not been severed and continues to afflict millions with avoidably worse health.

In fact, we can use Tiny Tim's experience of ill-health to draw a genealogy between the Cratchit's circumstances and millions of 'modern day Tiny Tims'. Rather than give a passing list, I look at two aspects of the Cratchit's poverty in detail: housing and employment.

Dickens describes the cramped quarters the Cratchit's live in, six people sharing four squat, smoke-filled rooms. Like Dickens' childhood home, the Cratchit's house is in London's Camden Town – a place the author would have associated with his own poverty and his father's imprisonment in debtor's prison. Later in life, Dickens described Camden as 'a complete bog of mud and filth with deep-cart ruts, wretched hovels, the doors blocked up with mud'.[5]

Today, housing continues to determine the health of millions. The English Housing Survey shows that 10 per cent of the UK's housing stock has what are known as 'Category 1 Hazards', including a disproportionate 600,000 homes in the private rented sector.[6] Category 1 hazards include serious and immediate dangers. There might be asbestos, a well-known cause of fatal lung conditions. There might also be serious mould or fungal growth – which can cause health problems for all but are particularly dangerous for those living with an existing respiratory condition like asthma. There could be carbon monoxide – the so called 'silent killer' – or other lethal substances, like lead or nitrogen dioxide.

Elsewhere, poor housing creates what are often wrongly seen as small discomforts, which can nevertheless snowball into serious health conditions. Just as Bob struggles for warmth in the opening scenes of Dicken's novella, millions today struggle to heat their homes in the UK. According to recent government data, an estimated 2.4 million households in England live in fuel poverty.[7] People who experience this are likely to try to 'put up' and cope the best they can. They might use their heating intermittently: for an hour a day, otherwise tolerating the cold. They may limit their lives to one or two rooms, which they can afford to heat more often. They may be forced to make a daily choice between heating or eating.[8]

Health consequences follow. One study by the Institute for Health Equity found that cold homes are linked to reduced weight gain in infants, asthma in young children, mental ill-health, increased incidence of flu, worse episodes of arthritis and (amongst old people) increased chance of heart attack, stroke, or chronic lung disease.[9] In any given year, tens of thousands of people die just because of excess cold – an epidemic on a similar scale to Covid, and one that is entirely preventable.[10]

As important as the quality of housing is the level of crowding within. Overcrowding affects 800,000 people today.[11] It is a plight almost exclusively experienced by people renting their homes – with 8 per cent of social renters and 6 per cent of private renters living in overcrowded conditions respectively.[12] From a health perspective, it is a key factor in the prevalence of Tuberculosis (TB) in this country. One study in London showed that when overcrowding increased by 1 per cent, TB infection rates also rose by 1 per cent.[13] Covid-19 was another infectious disease where cramped housing was tindering to rapid spread. Like many comparable diseases, Covid spreads more easily in indoor settings where people are in regular proximity. The government's Scientific Advisory Group for Emergencies (SAGE) not only identified a correlation between crowded houses and Covid-19 mortality but observed that link independently of the wider impacts of socio-economic deprivation.[14]

These figures come on the back of a litany of recent policy failures. In 2004, proposed legislation on a statutory overcrowding standard was touted but not introduced. A 2007 government pilot on overcrowding wasn't scaled. The Coalition government's 2011 Localism Act provided new tools to assess overcrowded housing but was reliant on the proactivity and good will of landlords, leaving renters at the unsympathetic whims of capital. Unsurprisingly, this meant little progress. New provisions on overcrowding proposed in the Lords stages of the 2016 *Housing and Planning Act* were withdrawn. All the while, homes continue to get smaller. The UK average new build is 76 square meters, the smallest in Europe[15] – and unaffordability continues to drive average occupancy of those homes up.

When compiled, one in seven of us live in unaffordable, insecure, or unsuitable homes – according to State of the Nation research by the National Housing Federation.[16] That's 8.4 million people: 3.6 million in overcrowded homes; 2.5 million in homes where they can't afford the mortgage or rent; 2.5 million living with parents or an ex-partner or friends; 1.7 million people in unsuitable housing – for instance, where they have a physical disability and can't get around or out their home; and 400,000 people at risk of homelessness. They have been let down by poor regulation, by a lack of social housing and by a government obsession with artificially inflating house prices. Like Tiny Tim, their access to health – regardless of their access to the NHS – is being sacrificed.

RACIALISED HEALTH INJUSTICE

In *A Christmas Carol*, Dickens does not go beyond poverty. But there is an onus on us to take the analysis further. Then and today, it's not only poverty that defines how health is distributed, it is also circumscribed by structures like race and gender.[17] The case study of work gives a clear insight into how racism, class and poverty interact to define the distribution of public health in modern Britain.

There is rich historic evidence showing how the nature of work impacts health. Beginning in 1967, the 'Whitehall study' of British civil servants looked at whether there was a link between grade of employment and mortality from disease.[18] The study tracked the health of thousands of British officials over a period of years, conclusively demonstrating that those in more junior roles had higher health risks and, in turn, a greater susceptibility to avoidable, premature mortality. Indeed, men in the lowest grades of work a three times higher mortality rate than men in the highest grades of work.

A follow up to the study published in *The Lancet* health journal in 1991 confirmed that there had been no reduction in the link between low-paid work and recommended 'more attention . . . be paid to the social environments, job design and the consequences of income inequality'.[19]

These might seem studies about class, but they are also absolutely studies in race – not least because the injustices of race and class can never be entirely separated. White people are more likely to have access to the well paid, fulfilling jobs that predict better health outcomes. In Whitehall today, ethnic minorities make up just 7–8 per cent of the senior civil service, but 12 per cent of civil servants overall and 11 per cent of the country's population.[20] That means that while Black people are taking up jobs that are essential to the functioning of the country and its public services, they are disproportionately exposed to work-related health risks, which impact both the quality and length of their life.

One of the experiences that best links the Cratchits with tens of thousands of Black people and families today is precariousness. Insecurity is a plight to the Cratchit family – Bob has little power in the face of his employer.[21] Today, the same sense of insecurity and lack of recourse is felt in many workplaces – but most of all, in the 'gig economy'.

In 2017, the government published the findings of the Taylor review into modern working practices. The review found that white workers were severely underrepresented in the gig economy. Indeed, just 68 per cent of gig economy workers described themselves as white British.[22] Elsewhere, it has been shown that Black workers are twice as likely to be on zero-hour contracts, as compared to white workers – driven in particular by a rise in Black women on zero-hour contracts, according to the TUC.[23]

Emerging research paints a bleak picture of the health consequences. A 2020 study for the Royal Society of Public Health's journal showed that workers paid on a 'piece rate' – that is pay per delivery made, job completed, or item produced – decreased workers' health, in comparison to salaried workers.[24] Piece rate is a growing tool to push productivity, not only in the gig economy, but in places like Amazon fulfilment factories. While not as obviously a health risk as heavy machinery, it is absolutely a high-impact occupational hazard.

Another study, led by Ursula Huws – professor of labour and globalisation at the Hertfordshire School of Business – identified some of the specific occupational health risks within gig economy roles.[25] These included physical risks – riding a bicycle to deliver food on busy London roads; sitting in a car for long periods;[26] a lack of proper health assessment; using equipment, like hot irons, without formal training.[27] They also included mental health risks – from waiting for work for hours; having to cancel social plans because a last minute shift came through; and feeling unable to say no to work, in case you're deactivated or deprioritised by your employer.[28]

These are all before we even bring in the question of pay. By the government's own figures, one in four in the gig economy earned less than £7.50 per hour in 2018 (the minimum wage that year).[29] Low pay is directly associated with poor health – both mental, including everything from stress to trauma, and physical, from respiratory problems through to heart disease.[30]

This can create a vicious cycle for those affected. One of the key barriers to secure, well-paid work is chronic illness or disability.[31] Poor work and low pay in turn create and sustain the conditions for worse health. It is only too easy to be caught in a cycle of reinforcing health and economic injustice. This is central to the inhumanity behind the Coalition government's austerity era Make Work Pay policies.[32]

While the gig economy comes with specific risks, the link between illness and racism is not just a problem of one sector. It infects the whole economy. Regardless of where they work, Black people are then more liable to experience a whole range of occupational health hazards within the workplace. In 2005, a study commissioned for the Health and Safety Executive concluded that – when looking at white people and people from minority ethnic backgrounds, of similar ages and roles – the latter were far more likely to experience stress and that the reasons for that stress was, explicitly, racial discrimination.[33] Seventeen years later, things haven't changed. The recent McGregor-Smith review documented that workplace disadvantages were still impacting the health of Black, Asian and minority ethnic people.[34]

When Dickens wrote his novella there were some instances of public health improvement underway, perhaps none more so than sanitation works to provide more people with clean water. Today, long working hours, bad bosses, receding workplace rights, poor private sector housing and precariousness are the equivalent of dirty water – killing hundreds of thousands each year, and sustaining disparities along the lines of race, occupation, class and material conditions.

Today's equivalent of the sanitation works would eliminate bad landlords, bad bosses and poverty.

WHY HAS NOTHING CHANGED?

There is clearly value in compiling the latest evidence. But I'm not the first person to highlight these drivers of poor health. In 1980, the *Black Report* was a landmark in establishing structural drivers of health inequality.[35] In 2010, Michael Marmot's report *Fair Society Healthy Lives* established a whole host of 'social determinants of health' beyond what is in the scope of a medical health service.[36]

And while these reports stand out as seminal, even they don't constitute particularly revolutionary additions to overall knowledge. The first national Whitehall department for health – the Ministry of Health, set up in 1919 – contained functions well beyond hospitals. It oversaw National Insurance, the Poor Law, local government, community planning, housing and environmental health.[37] That is, it demonstrated a fundamental understanding – and a far better one than often seen today – of the need for a holistic definition of health.

Political and policy inaction on poverty and health – or racism and health, gender and health, transphobia and health – hasn't been enabled by a paucity in our knowledge. There are two more important reasons that good public health research has not been translated into truly radical policy change. First, the continued dominance of the idea of personal responsibility for our health, which constrains the scope for state-led interventions. Second, a lack of totemic ideas around which advocates of an alternative can coalesce.

We can return to *A Christmas Carol* for illuminating commentary on the idea of personal responsibility. It's the politics of choice for the unreformed Ebenezer Scrooge – one that allows him to justify his miserliness; the hawkishness of his business practices; and the brutality of his employment standards.

"Are there no Prisons?" asked Scrooge.

"Plenty of prisons," said the gentleman, laying down the pen again.

"And the Union workhouses?" demanded Scrooge. "Are they still in operation?"

"They are. Still," returned the gentleman, "I wish I could say they were not."

"The Treadmill and the Poor Law are in full vigour, then?" said Scrooge.

"Both very busy, sir."

"Oh, I was afraid, from what you said at first, that something had occurred to stop them in their useful course," said Scrooge.

"Under the impression that they scarcely furnish Christian cheer of mind or body to the multitude," returned the gentleman, "a few of us are endeavouring to raise a fund to buy the Poor some meat and drink, and means of warmth. We choose this time, because it is a time, of all others, when Want is keenly felt, and Abundance rejoices. What shall I put you down for?"

"Nothing!" Scrooge replied.

"You wish to be anonymous?"

"I wish to be left alone," said Scrooge. "Since you ask me what I wish gentlemen, that is my answer. I don't make merry myself at Christmas, and I can't afford to make idle people merry. I help support the establishments I have mentioned: they cost enough: and those who are badly off must go there."

"Many can't go there; and many would rather die."

"If they would rather die," said Scrooge, "they had better do it, and decrease the surplus population. Besides – excuse me – I don't know that."

"But you might know it," observed the gentleman.

"It is not my business," Scrooge returned. "It's enough for a man to understand his own business, and not to interfere with other people's. Mine occupies me constantly. Good afternoon, gentleman."

'Decrease the surplus population' is a shocking utterance. But it is the last few lines that are, perhaps, more telling. They expose Scrooge's fundamental belief in personal responsibility and self-interest in determining health, wellbeing and welfare. Those unable to independently improve their own lot must deal with the consequences.

That this point of view appears in an early-Victorian novella might imply it's an antiquated belief. But it remains dominant today, and its articulation can be found among politicians on both the political left and political right.

In 2018, former Secretary of State for Health and Social Care Matt Hancock said: 'We need to do far more to personally take responsibility for our own health'. His 2018 green paper *Prevention is Better than Cure* took the theme further.[38] It focused on 'empowering people to manage their own physical and mental health needs' – a viewpoint that makes health about individual agency, not social or economic circumstance. Boris Johnson has put it in more 'on the nose' terms – penning a *Telegraph* op-ed in 2004 entitled: 'Face it, it's All Your Own Fat Fault'.[39] While in 2004, then Labour's Secretary of State for Health John Reid told the *Guardian*:

> I just do not think the worst problem on our sink estate by any means is smoking, but it is an obsession of the learned middle class . . . what enjoyment does a 21-year-old single mother of three living in a council estate get? The only enjoyment sometimes they have is to have a cigarette.[40]

Reid's argument poses as the more empathetic but remains a caricature of people wedded to the same politics of civil liberty and opposition to state intervention that underpins the ideas communicated by the political right.

FREE SCHOOL MEALS

More recently, debate around free school meal provisions has provided another case study in the power of the personal responsibility paradigm. Reacting to campaign work by Manchester United footballer Marcus Rashford, Kevin Hollinrake MP wrote: 'where they can it's a parent's job to feed their children'. Ben Bradley MP took his argument further:

> Mad world we live in where saying that parents are responsible for feeding their children is now seen as wildly offensive and controversial. Dare I say that a long-term degradation of personal responsibility is part of the problem here? You don't fix poverty with freebies!![41]

There is now formal research that shows the dominance of personal responsibility in public health policy. In January 2021, a study published in *The Milbank Quarterly* by Dolly Theis and Martin White reviewed interventions on the issue of obesity – an area where personal responsibility discourse is particularly prominent – between 1992 and 2020. Their research found that, firstly, (cross-party) policies overwhelmingly make high demands of individual agency and behaviour change. Crucially, they also find that where policies *seem* to break with this and suggest a more interventionist approach, they are overwhelmingly formulated in a way that 'does not readily lead to implementation'.[42]

This is all to expose a major friction that sits at the heart of health policy in twenty-first century Britain. When it comes to medical treatment, we have a system formulated on collective responsibility whereby we all come together to share the cost of extending a comprehensive, modern healthcare system to everyone.

By contrast, the status quo when it comes to public health before a diagnosis is a viewpoint that early, avoidable, or unfortunate cases of illness are a consequence of bad behaviour – rather than the violence of poverty or racism engraved upon our bodies. We are a country that is happy with state intervention to treat the misfortune of illness, but not to address the conditions in which illness occurs.

CHALLENGING PERSONAL RESPONSIBILITY

Evidently, personal responsibility for our health is a tempting notion. In my own work, I hear it surprisingly frequently from people on the left, as well as people on the political right – including at times from democratic socialists who would never openly subscribe to meritocracy.

Just as with developed leftist rebuttals to meritocracy, the most powerful counter is to focus on some of the highly suspect conclusions that personal responsibility implicitly relies on. Namely, that it demands that we believe that Black people, working class people, people living in the North or people in insecure work all experience health inequalities because of a common moral failure.

Take the town of Blackpool. Residents of this seaside resort are about twice as likely as others in England to be admitted to hospital for intentional self-harm. They are also about twice as likely to be admitted to hospital for an alcohol-related health condition. Teenagers living there have a one in three chance of becoming pregnant before the age of 18, compared to a one in six chance in the rest of England. People are more likely to suffer a violent crime, and twice as likely to be hospitalised by that violence than in the rest of England. The obesity rate is twice the England average.

Compare that to Wokingham, a pretty market town in Berkshire, South England. Here, life expectancy is two and a half years higher than the England average. It's far, far less likely you'll die of a serious illness like cancer or heart disease before age 75. There are fewer serious injuries on its roads. Fewer children live in low-income families, the homeless rate is very low and hospital admissions for violence are far rarer than the country's average. If you live in Wokingham, then it is not impossible that you'll experience bad health – or even worse health than a friend or family member in Blackpool. But it is much, much less likely, on every single count.[43]

Inescapably, the personal responsibility hypothesis concludes that people in Blackpool are subject to some moral failure not often found among the people of Wokingham. It does not and cannot entertain the idea that it might be down to the fact Blackpool is one of the most deprived parts of the country. Or the fact that Blackpool's tourist economy has been hit hard in recent decades. Or that its experience of deindustrialisation has hit jobs and communities. Or that 40 per cent of private sector dwellings in Blackpool have been classed as non-decent.[44] Or that austerity has disproportionately hit its local authority and public health budgets. Or that people in Blackpool must contend with fewer jobs, lower incomes and worse education outcomes than people elsewhere.[45]

Personal responsibility is a paradigm with no room for empathy or mitigating factors.

Personal responsibility as a notion can even have negative clinical consequences. This finding has been seen particularly clearly around lung cancer. Research shows that experience of stigma among lung cancer patients – linked to its strong association with tobacco use – can cause anxiety, depression and the severity of physical symptoms.[46] Significantly, this impacts both lung cancer patients who smoked heavily, but also lung cancer patients who have never smoked. Personal responsibility is a health hazard in its own right.[47]

The opportunity offered by the social justice frontier is an expansion of leftist health principles to address the drivers of health need currently outside the remit of the NHS. The opportunity can be conceptualised by thinking about the elements of health that Nye Bevan did *not* include in his conception of a comprehensive health service.

A simple conception of a 'health pathway' might run as follows:

- The conditions in which we live: This covers the variables that define our life and lifestyle, and covers broad social factors like experience of poverty, income, education, employment, relationships, childhood events, low pay, or homelessness.
- A direct cause: Something puts us at causal risk of ill health (smoking, poor diet, lack of exercise, dangerous hobbies, alcohol or drug addiction, low income, problem debt, hazardous housing).
- A symptom emerges: We notice something wrong. Our heart is racing. Our breath is short. We have a pain, or lump, or bump.
- We seek help: In the UK, there are two main access points. First, a General Practitioner, who provides a gateway into the health system itself. Secondly, Accident and Emergency, when the need is more pressing.
- We get diagnosed: Our illness is identified, either by a physical examination, some medical equipment, or so forth.
- We get treatment: ranging from physiotherapy to pain relief, antibiotics, medicine, or surgery.

When he created the National Health Service, Bevan did not create a health service that covered the entirety of this pathway. The NHS intervenes about halfway through – somewhere between the point we notice a symptom and the point we receive a formal diagnosis.[48] That leaves a whole region of space where our health is not supported by a publicly run, universal system. This is where his principles – universalising the best, free at the point of delivery, based on need, funded by taxation and available to all – are most dearly needed.

THE UNIVERSAL PUBLIC HEALTH SERVICE

The crucial question is this: could the NHS's principles of collectivism and state intervention be extended to social inequality? Can we extend the NHS's brilliance to preventing illness – to taking on the conditions that make people sick – rather than just treating it? The answer is yes, with bold ambition and political will – through a new **Universal Public Health Service**.

In fact, the country has a (tiny) version of this already in place. Local public health services are currently delivered through a ring-fenced grant – 'the public health grant' – and overseen by a Director of Public Health in each local authority. These services are remarkable for being both incredibly effective and extremely cost efficient. To give an example – putting a single pound into local sexual health service budgets comes with a return on investment of £11. For every £1 spent locally on preventing children from starting smoking, we can recoup £15 worth of benefits.[49] One study concluded that public health services are 'three to four times more productive' in producing health benefits than NHS healthcare services.[50]

Despite this, the budget for the public health grant has faced severe cuts during the last decade. My research shows that the budget has been cut by a quarter since 2013/14. Worse, those cuts have almost exclusively come from the poorest parts of the country. The ten least deprived local authorities in England have shouldered just £1 in every £46 cut from local services, while the ten most deprived have put up £1 in every £7.[51]

These are services designed to save the NHS money and, most importantly, avoid people experiencing life changing diagnoses, wherever they can be avoided. Unsurprisingly, the cost of cutting such services was keenly felt during Covid-19 – a disease that thrived in places where underlying health conditions were most common. My analysis has shown that areas that saw the highest mortality rates in the first wave of the pandemic had experienced local public health budget cuts three and a half times greater than areas where Covid mortality was lowest.[52]

Even at their peak, our public health service has never had anything like the firepower needed to fully prevent the vast amount of avoidable ill-health people experience today. Between national and local services, the total budget comes to about £4 billion a year – a pittance on which to run anything like a comprehensive public health system. £4 billion is the equivalent of just 2–2.5 per cent of everything spent on health and social care in England.

A Universal Public Health Service (UPHS) would be about scaling our ambition on state-led public health services by an order of magnitude. It would take forward a very simple principle: if we are willing to collectively pay for cancer treatment when someone gets sick, we should be willing to pay for a social intervention that – based on the evidence – would prevent someone from receiving that diagnosis. Not only would this improve our total stock of health, and make a huge contribution to health justice, it would make our overall health spending far more efficient and take huge strain off the National Health Service in the years and decades to come.

A few models could provide the foundation for this endeavour. Research that aims to identify the root causes of poor health tends to include the following:

- Access to high quality, holistic education
- Access to healthy, sustainable diet
- Good quality employment, pay and occupational health standards
- Financial wellbeing
- Access to good, affordable housing
- Social relationships and community ties
- Access to utilities, such as heating, clean water, and internet
- Fair distribution of income and wealth

In 2021, I published research using the ONS' Health Index that showed – in the most recent data – the most consistent predictors of good health in places included: 1) what happens in our early years and school years; 2) levels of income and wealth inequality; 3) rates and experiences of poverty, particularly in childhood; and 4) the access children have to healthy diets.[53] This indicates where gains can immediately be secured, and where the UPHS should prioritise.

In its first iteration, a Universal Public Health Service could cover each of these. In doing so, it need not be 'one-size-fits-all'. The mission of the Universal Public Health Service should be a) creating an evidence base of social interventions that demonstrably improves health (i.e., equivalent to the medical breakthroughs that provide new drugs); b) allowing local public health experts to seek out need in their local communities (equivalent to diagnosis) and c) ensuring the resources are in place to address those needs, whatever these may be (the equivalent to allocating treatment). In every case, this should be relational – decisions should be made with, not for, people. No-one should be compelled to accept help, in the same way they are not compelled to accept medical treatment.[54] Specific service delivery should be led primarily from places, rather than from Whitehall – recognising that there are very different social priorities, even in places with very similar health profiles. And funding should be heavily weighted towards the most deprived parts of the country, recognising differences like those we've already discussed between Wokingham and Blackpool.

Below I outline what a core offer for such a service could look like when first formed.

Prescription 1: Equal Education for All

Good education is a vital foundation for good, lifelong health. There are some ways where the overlap between health and education is obvious: sex education; a progressive approach to teaching about drugs and alcohol; a school environment that values relationships; the provision of counselling and mental health support. This can all provide a strong basis for a healthy life.

But education that is not 'health education' is just as important (if not more). In 2010, Professor Sir Michael Marmot concluded his report on health inequalities by observing that:

> Inequalities in educational outcomes affect physical and mental health, as well as income, employment and quality of life . . . To achieve equity from the start, investment in early years is crucial. However, maintaining the reduction of inequalities across the gradient also requires a sustained commitment to children and young people through the years of education.[55]

Elsewhere, education disparities have been linked to very tangible health injustices. Children with the best education are estimated to have a life expectancy four years higher than those with the worst, by the time both are aged 30.[56]

The universality of the UK's education system has never been more at threat. One of the clearest examples of this are the rising rates of exclusion from school. Having fallen at the start of the century, the last decade has seen a perilous rise, with 8,000 children excluded permanently from school in 2018/19. In the same period, over half a million children had a fixed-period exclusion – a rise of 25,000 in a year.[57]

Overwhelmingly, these exclusions impact people from minority ethnic backgrounds. People who identify as part of the traveller community have a one in five chance of experiencing an exclusion; Black Caribbean children have a one in ten chance, and white British children a one in twenty chance.[58] Those children are more likely to experience severe psychological distress in the immediate aftermath of the event.[59]

Elsewhere, there is the pernicious practice of 'off-rolling' – whereby a school removes a pupil without recourse to a formal 'permanent exclusion' (i.e. by pressuring the parent to remove their child).[60] In 2019, as many as 49,101 students simply disappeared from school roll. A disproportionate number are from 'Black ethnic backgrounds' according to figures from the Education Policy Institute.[61]

Exclusion is not guaranteed to impact the long-term health of children. But it does immediately and significantly increase the risk of worse long-term health outcomes. Beyond exclusions, there are severe attainment gaps across and within our schools. By the time they finish their GCSEs at age 15 or 16, the most disadvantaged children will be a year and a half of learning behind their peers.[62] The attainment gap is only likely to widen in the aftermath of Covid-19. Research before the pandemic showed that time away from schools – like the summer holidays – widens the education gap between the most and least affluent children.[63]

The impact of 2020/1 school closures, combined with insufficient catch-up funding, is therefore very likely to cause significant inequality.[64]

One of the key levers intended to address educational inequality in England is the 'pupil premium' – through which extra funding is allocated to schools serving eligible children. In principle the policy is a good one – it allocates resources to the poorest in society, at a point early enough in their life to make a major difference. In practice, however, the premium has not narrowed the attainment gap.

The problem is one of coverage and of scale. Currently, a state secondary school will receive £955 a year – less than £3 a day – to address the impact of deprivation on a child's education.[65] A primary school will receive a little more: about £1,345 per student, or just £4 a day. For even these small sums of money, there is no mechanism to reliably ensure the funding benefits the child who needs it. Indeed, secondary schools in the most deprived parts of England saw their budgets cut by about 13 per cent between 2009/10 and 2019/20 – compared to a 9 per cent average cut – making pupil premiums little more than lip service.[66]

It makes for a woeful comparison to the advantages the most affluent parents can provide their children. Average private school fees now stand at £17,000 per year.[67] That might then be topped up further – through school trip fees, sports equipment, extra tuition, after school clubs, or musical instruments. Put in these terms, it's unsurprising that the evidence shows wealthy children outperform talented children in the educational system.[68]

Given how conclusive the evidence is on the link between education and health throughout our lives, any lack of sufficient education investment is a classic case of short-sightedness. It makes little sense if we simply pick up the tab in healthcare costs later. For that reason, the Universal Public Health Service should introduce a bigger and more targeted pupil premium package, based on giving the most disadvantaged children access to private school advantages within the state sector.[69]

Delivery could work as follows. A local public health team could work with schools in their area to identify where educational needs are greatest. They could then work with children and their families and carers to establish what their priorities and ambitions are. Then the public health professional could put in place a package of financial support that revolutionises that child's education. By working alongside families, teachers and school administrators – to create a personalised and funded education plan – the issue of targeting the support at individual children would be immediately corrected.

In terms of resourcing the prescription, tripling the resource available – and ensuring it is far better targeted – would revolutionise the ability of education to provide every child the best foundation for a healthy life. At an outlay of £7.2 billion per year, public health professionals would have around £4,000 available to support the education of our most deprived primary school children. That early investment would be recouped not only through healthier adults, who make less use of the health service, but through a stronger, fairer economy.[70] The interventions funding through the premium need not be aggressively focused on attainment. It might be that money is not best targeted at extra tuition, but at providing counselling, speech and language therapy, nutritious lunches. The latter better align with what parents and children currently think schools most need.[71]

The importance of holistic opportunities suggest we should take this prescription one step further. Children in the most affluent families have access to any number of hobbies – music, sport and art. Again, this is good for health. Not only does participation in extra-curricular activities help academic outcomes, but they also immediately boost a child's health. The most recent evidence shows that ability to participate in an extra-curricular hobby increased levels of optimism and life satisfaction, and reduced depressive symptoms and levels of anxiety.[72]

For £720 million per year, the state could provide the Universal Public Health Service with the means to 'prescribe' every child on free school meals a hobby of their choice – and recoup those costs through better childhood mental health. This would clearly be timely. A childhood mental health crisis is one of the clearest legacies of Covid-

19. One indicative study found a 44 per cent increase in symptoms of depression and a 26 per cent increase in PTSD among eleven–twelve-year-olds during just the first national lockdown.[73] While it is important the NHS is there for them, public health interventions like this one could stop that need from either developing or worsening.

Prescription 2: Nutritious, Free Meals to End Food Poverty

In October 2020, the Queen's birthday honours included an MBE for twenty-two-year-old Marcus Rashford. Earlier in the year, he had won a significant victory on his campaign for free holiday meals for school children. The award of the MBE did not put any halt to his campaigning. Just days later, he restarted his campaign in reaction to a decision by the UK government not to extend school meals to April 2021 in England. Scotland, Wales and Northern Ireland had, by contrast, chosen to maintain provision.

Food insecurity is a major and multifaceted problem in Britain today. Even before Covid-19.3 million children were at risk of holiday hunger, which can cause severe emotional distress, including trauma; can lead to physical health problems because of malnutrition; and can lead to worse educational outcomes, the importance of which we have just covered.[74] But in modern Britain, the consequences of food insecurity also go beyond hunger. A combination of rising prices for healthy food – and an increase in the accessibility of cheap, unhealthy food – means obesity, hunger and malnutrition often go hand in hand. Around two thirds of adults are overweight or obese, childhood obesity has reached record levels, both adult and child obesity is more common among people living in poverty, and has direct causal links to cancer, coronary heart disease and Type II diabetes.[75]

A Universal Public Health Service would allow us to implement a very simple solution: free nutritious food, for everyone that needs it, when they need it. The evidence behind giving people healthy food, when they can't afford it, is compelling. It has been shown to improve security, quality of life and diet.[76] It simultaneously tackles hunger and obesity.[77] It is nothing short of a silver-bullet when it comes to childhood health.

When implemented, free nutritious food schemes have often been highly successful. A scheme called Rose Vouchers run in several local authorities throughout the UK, has shown some remarkable outcomes. The scheme runs as follows: someone in the children's services sector identifies a child or family in need; that child's family is given £3 to £6 per week to spend in open air fruit and veg markets; the family gets better food security and local businesses are boosted. Formal evaluation has shown:

- Children and families using the scheme were happier and healthier
- Families using the vouchers ate less unhealthy food like takeaways
- Families using the vouchers ate more fruit and vegetables[78]

The Universal Public Health Service could simply scale this example of local innovation – by providing a universal healthy food prescription service.

There is a growing movement in support of this idea. In Summer 2020, the IPPR released a cost proposal for a food subsidy of £21, for all children at risk of food poverty. As well as providing better health, food security is also beneficial for planetary health.[79] Calls for a healthy food scheme are part of the final conclusions from the landmark Commission for Environmental Justice.[80] This link between good health and climate will be discussed in more detail in Chapter 5.

Prescription 3: A Right to Healthy Housing

This chapter has already covered the public health consequences of housing in modern Britain in some detail. The relationship between housing and poor health was only accentuated by Covid, as many with insufficient space or poor-quality housing were forced to stay inside for very long periods of time – and to convert their living space, simultaneously, into school and office.

The case of homelessness was particularly acute. In the wake of the Covid-19 outbreak, the government launched the 'Everyone in' operation – providing hotel and emergency accommodation to those who needed it. Though not perfect, the scheme was widely praised by campaigners and charities. It provided proof that homelessness and rough sleeping could be addressed if there is the will to act decisively. However, the political will proved short lived. The second lockdown in the Winter of 2020/1 came without a return of the everyone-in policy – leaving homeless people exposed to a combination of the elements and the pandemic. This was a political choice.

The health consequences of poor housing cannot be disaggregated from the stock and quality of affordable social housing. The number of people living in social homes halved between 1980 and 2010, and has continued to fall since.[81] This has meant many more people entering the private rented sector, which is often unsustainably expensive. According to Trust for London, average rent currently equals 46.4 per cent of the median pre-tax pay in the capital per cent of the average household income – and 24.1 per cent in the rest of the country.[82] Such extensive costs are one of the dominant drivers of poverty, particularly in-work poverty, across the country.[83]

In their outline of a Universal Basic Services offer, a team from University College London explored what a radical upgrade in social housing stock would look like. Their modelling estimated that meeting needs in the UK would require 1.5 million new social houses – provided rent free.[84]

While their case is not anchored in public health per se, the availability of this stock would be revolutionary from a public health perspective. 1.5 million homes would allow the public health service to provide alternative accommodation for those with severe public health hazards in their homes, where a fix cannot otherwise be properly offered. It would provide, immediately, for the 220,000 people experiencing 'core homelessness' in 2019 – i.e., those sleeping on the streets or stuck in temporary accommodation.[85] And it could be used to significantly alleviate the experience of over-crowding experienced by hundreds of thousands.[86]

The Universal Public Health Service could provide housing on a social prescription model relatively easily. Local directors of public health would simply need to identify levels of need in their area, and work with national bodies to commission adequate supplies of 'public health housing'. Once built, public health teams would work with local government to allocate housing to those who need it.

Where homelessness has rocketed in the UK since 2010, other countries have managed to make progress against its proliferation. Finland has seen a drop of 35 per cent by using a simple scheme. They give houses to people who need them, through a 'housing first' model. While the scheme initially only targeted long-term homeless people, a subsequent programme has included prevention of homelessness in the remit. Finland is the only country in Europe to have reduced homelessness since the financial crash.[87] By way of comparison, UK homelessness rose by 134 per cent between 2009 and 2015.[88]

Homelessness is not the only health challenge related to housing that this prescription would target, but this is indicative of the idea that the scheme can work. Moreover, it demonstrates how, while evidently not cheap, delivering health improvement through social justice should be a lynchpin of a Universal Public Health Service.

Prescription 4: Ending the Health Costs of Utility Poverty

Utilities are evidently a prime candidate for a 'free at the point of delivery based on need' approach. First, they tend towards monopoly – one national grid, one owner of regional water pipes. This makes it easy to exclude people in the interest of profit. Second, consumers do not have any choice about needing the product. It is not a consumer luxury; it is a human need.

Almost all utilities can accentuate poor health and the conditions that lead to it. I've already talked about heating, but electricity can be another source of significant stress and need across UK households. The price of power has been rising over time. For example, between 2004 and 2010, electricity prices rose by 44 per cent in real terms – vastly outstripping the cost of living.[89] Those on pay as you go meters are the most likely to find themselves cut off from power, pay the most, and are more likely to be struggling financially anyway. It is a factor in embedding poverty, more broadly defined.

Within the bracket of utilities, digital exclusion must also be considered a clear public health priority. As of 2018, 5.3 million adults in the UK still experienced exclusion from the internet.[90] The Centre for Economics and Business Research, an independent economic forecasting and analysis company, has shown that such exclusion comes with tangible impacts. People who are digitally excluded earn between 3 and 10 per cent less than they otherwise would; they are more likely to be unemployed; they likely have a higher cost of living (online shopping is 13 per cent cheaper on average); they miss opportunities to connect with the community; and they spend longer on routine actions (such as online vs. physical banking).[91]

These are impacts that a Universal Public Health Service should concern itself with on a health and quality of life basis. Such unnecessary and avoidable lost earnings, lost employment potential and increased basic costs will impact life chances. Reviews of the evidence have found a conclusive link between money and ill health – both physical and mental.[92]

Digital exclusion also bars people from a range of direct NHS services. The NHS is making an inevitable move towards digital technology. This was accelerated during the pandemic – with a massive reduction in physical GP appointments, a shift to electronic bookings, a large amount of health information moving online and the introduction of large-scale health apps.

Each of these is amenable to policy – namely, giving everyone who needs it free access to the core resources of twenty-first century life.

Prescription 5: Prescribing Against Low Pay and Low Hope

Work has been a consistent focus in this chapter's exploration of non-medical drivers of health injustice. It would be amiss if a founding offer from the Universal Public Health Service did not offer an intervention aimed at employment.

Simply having a job is not a predictor of the conditions needed to live a healthy life in Britain today. I have already covered occupational health, but in-work poverty is a key problem, too. Over one in four households found to be homeless or under threat of homelessness contained one or more people in work, as of 2019.[93] 56 per cent of people (seven in ten children) in poverty in 2018 lived in a working household, compared with 39 per cent 20 years ago.[94] One in seven food bank users are employed or live with someone who is employed.[95]

From a health perspective, this creates a clear case for increased access to training and adult education. More obviously, it makes the case for universal cash payments, provided to those whose income would put them at risk of poverty – and the health harms that have been detailed throughout this chapter.

The skills component could embody an idea that has already begun to generate momentum – a 'skills wallet'. In the 2019 general election, one of the headline pledges from the Liberal Democrats was a 'skills wallet' – providing £4,000 for training and further education at age 25, £3,000 at age 40 and £3,000 at age 55. The costing came to £1.9 billion a year – which the party said could be covered many times over by reversing cuts in Corporation Tax since 2016.[96]

Translating the idea to public health interventions would require some adjustments. It would be available for those who need it, as a prescription against a lack of further education opportunities suppressing their health and creating substantial health injustices. The specifics of the training – where it takes place, at what level and what aspirations it would support could be decided in partnership between the people who receive it and the public health teams who administer it.

The cash payment component of this prescription would essentially constitute a public health minimum income guarantee – designed to bring people up to an independently assessed 'Healthy Income Standard'. This could be based, directly, on existing conceptions of a Minimum income Guarantee.

The basis for the intervention can be drawn from international trials, such as in Finland. There, a pilot scheme saw 2,000 unemployed people given 560 euros per month, with no conditions on how the money would be used. Evaluation shows significant improvements in financial well-being, mental health, cognitive functioning and levels of confidence in the future. Economic security improved. A small increase in employment was observed (compared to those on Finland's existing benefits scheme). Poverty, bureaucracy and administration costs all decreased. The conditions for a healthy, high quality of life were in place and the model was deemed sustainable, indicating it could be taken and translated from an economic intervention to a public health prescription.[97]

The Finnish pilot has often been derided exactly because the impact on employment was not large. The evaluation records that:

> The employment effects of the basic income experiment were measured for the period from November 2017 to October 2018. The employment rate for basic income recipients improved slightly more during this period than for the control group.[98]

This is an unfair ground on which to dismiss the experiment. Until this pilot, UBI had been avoided because it might actively harm employment – by weakening incentives to work. A small improvement in employment amongst the UBI group is, in some ways, a remarkable departure from the previously accepted orthodoxy.

Of course, such public health-led state interventions in the welfare system should not be designed in a way that encourages employers to simply pay their employees less. This is already a dynamic in the make-up of the UK's welfare system. Research from Citizens UK in 2014 found that the taxpayer tops up wages by £11 billion a year – and that low pay amongst just the four big supermarkets (Tesco, Asda, Sainsburys and Morrisons) cost £1 billion a year in tax credits and extra benefit payments. This kind of situation, which essentially subsidises bad corporate behaviours, can be avoided. Ensuring that the public health interventions here do not simply fuel health exploitation at the hands of capital is the explicit focus of the next chapter.

A SILVER BULLET FOR SUSTAINABILITY

In the twentieth century, we experienced a golden age in health. Our life expectancy rose rapidly, as new medical advances beat back long-standing plights on the nation's health. Today, we are doubling down on that same model of care. However, the interventions that are likely to deliver real progress today will probably require a fundamental change in focus from the established model of twentieth-century health interventions. In justifying the idea of social interventions, Alan Logan and colleagues argued in 2019 that:

> [E]ach person/community should be viewed as a biological manifestation of accumulated experiences (and choices) made within the dynamic, political, economic and cultural ecosystems that comprise their total life history. This requires an understanding that powerful forces operate within these ecosystems; marketing and neoliberal forces push an exclusive 'personal responsibility view of health – blaming the individual and deflecting from the large-scale influence that maintain health inequalities and threaten planetary health.[99]

They highlight exactly how personal responsibility in health – like meritocracy in the workplace, individualism in society, consumer-sovereignty in economics – functions. It supports a small-state view, obscuring the influences of vested interests. As we'll explore in the next chapter, it particularly obscures the vested interests of capital.

This made Covid-19 very difficult for the political right. As an infectious disease pandemic, it made it very hard to maintain a personal responsibility paradigm – not least, because the link between who took the 'irresponsible' action and who suffered the consequences was broken. For a small period of time, the government was pushed towards otherwise unimaginable public health interventions such as the furlough scheme and 'Everyone In' – at the kind of scale demanded by the wider, non-pandemic health reality of rising chronic disease. Sadly, they were schemes limited in decisiveness, scope and duration, as ideology adapted and reasserted itself.

The right will now look to do three things. Firstly, they will suggest 'never again' on public health. Second, they will argue that the big state does not and cannot work in the face of health challenges. They will, wrongly, put lockdown at the heart of the coming years of health and NHS strain – when, in fact, it massively reduced the impact of a Covid pandemic fuelled by austerity, neoliberalism and rising inequality. Third, they will look to exceptionalize Covid-19, as entirely different from chronic non-infectious ('non-communicable') diseases – to avoid big public health interventions against major health challenges becoming the norm.

They are wrong on each count. Overwhelmingly, public health interventions protected our health and our long-term NHS capacity in the face of the lack of resilience discussed in Chapter One. Moreover, we can absolutely view non-communicable diseases as a pandemic with very similar dynamics. Only, rather than passing through air droplets, they are transmitted socially, across places and generations, through the unjust structure of our society and the lack of material conditions that still afflict millions. In this light, we need schemes to collectivise risk and meet the health challenge at the same scale as lockdowns and furlough. And fortunately, in this case we do not need more national shutdowns – far more palatably, we need a Universal Public Health Service.

3

The Economic Frontier

In the 1940s, tobacco companies were busy pushing the idea that their products came with a host of wonderful health benefits. One Lucky Strike poster declared '20,679 Physicians say "Luckies are less irritating" . . . your throat's protection against irritation, against cough [sic]'. Camels, a leading brand of the R.J. Reynolds Tobacco Company, went with a similar line: 'More doctors smoke Camels than any other cigarette'.[1]

Major advertising campaigns were a key factor in rising smoking rates in the first half of the twentieth century. Prior to this, evidence suggests that lung cancer had been a comparatively rare diagnosis.[2] Fewer people received a cancer diagnosis at all, and lung cancer made up a smaller proportion of these diagnoses. This changed sharply in the ensuing decades, with one study of men in America showing an increase in prevalence from about 5 in every 100,000 to about 75 in every 100,000 between 1930 and 1990.[3]

The changing epidemiology of such a lethal disease drove an urgent search for the cause, with tobacco a key suspect. Through the 1940s and 50s, the case against tobacco became irrefutable. In the UK, a decisive piece of research was released by Richard Doll and Austin Bradford Hill in 1954. Through a survey of smoking habits among NHS doctors,[4] they presented damning proof of a causal relationship between the number of cigarettes smoked and lung cancer risk.[5]

From here, momentum built. In 1962 the Royal College of Physicians made a landmark recommendation of a major programme of tobacco control; in 1964, the US Surgeon General published a report arguing for the same; and in 1965, the UK government took its first regulatory steps, with a ban on television tobacco adverts.[6]

Despite some public health wins, it's hard to conclude that the industry has been anything other than remarkably successful in defending its product. Big tobacco remains a global powerhouse. The legal tobacco market has sales worth approximately $820 billion per annum, thanks to the 5.7 trillion cigarettes consumed per year by the 19 per cent of the world's population who smoke.[7] In the UK, the tobacco industry attests to tax payments worth over £10 billion per year, employment of thousands and an economic contribution worth over £2 billion/annum.[8]

Moreover, big tobacco continues to post financial results that defy the widely held assumption that it has become an unsustainable industry and will simply cease to exist as consumers and policy makers react to its harms. In May 2021, Imperial Brands – formerly, Imperial Tobacco: the world's fifth biggest tobacco company – reported a £3.6 billion increase in revenue. Finance experts Hargreaves & Lansdown put this above-expectations result down to 'strong pricing and product mix'.[9] Faithful shareholders were rewarded with an increased dividend payment.

Vintage years were toasted elsewhere, too, with British and American Tobacco highlighting 2020 as 'a strong one for BAT's global business'[10] and Phillip Morris International claiming an 'outstanding delivery by the organization'.[11]

Such excellent end of year financial reports translates to disastrous health consequences. In the UK, around 7 million adults smoke and, according to Public Health England, around 78,000 deaths per year are directly attributable to smoking in England alone.[12] That is more deaths than were caused by Covid in England and Wales throughout 2020.[13] Many more people are diagnosed with a serious, long-term smoking related illness such as chronic obstructive pulmonary disease (COPD).[14] Perhaps most alarming is evidence that shows tobacco use is the single largest cause of health inequalities, accounting for as much as half of the difference in 'amendable mortality'[15] between the most and least deprived communities in the country.[16] By 2030, it is predicted that global tobacco deaths will break 8 million per year.[17] This is assuming that Covid-19 does not lead to a smoking boom – which is far from certain. The number of young adults who smoke in England rose by a quarter in 2020, according to research by University College London and the University of Sheffield.[18]

A slow decline in the UK and Western markets has given big tobacco the time it needed to build a sustainable global presence. It is amongst the biggest benefactors, and most aggressive utilisers, of globalisation. Indeed, despite the industry's negative image in much of Europe and North America, systematic reviews show they have actively positioned themselves as good corporate citizens elsewhere.[19] Taking the global view, the industry now looks as big and strong as it ever has.

At times, the tobacco industry has been able to use some unbelievable methods to avoid regulation. In some cases, they've gone as far as manufacturing and sustaining black markets, by oversupplying cheap tobacco to neighbours of regulating countries in an attempt to undercut their efforts.[20] In one case, reacting to a ban on cigarette imports in Vietnam, British and American Tobacco set up a Cambodia outfit to smuggle cigarettes into the nation – using legal trade flows to mask their illegal smuggling operation.[21] This bypassed legitimate tobacco control policies, for profit – and allowed BAT, whose role in the contraband was not known, to point to the presence of a black market in lobbying the Vietnamese government to open up a legitimate market. After six years, Vietnam caved and rowed back on their tobacco control approach, demonstrating the power of capital to profit from health can defy even national sovereignty.[22]

THE 'BAD EGG' FALLACY

The severity of the health impacts of extravagantly unhealthy industries like big tobacco – and the aggressive tactics used by its lobbyists, at home and abroad – often mean it's highlighted as an exceptional, rather than archetypal, case of health exploitation. This exceptionalisation of a small number of industries in public health advocacy is something I call the **bad egg fallacy**.

The bad egg fallacy views the exploitation of our health for profit by the very worst businesses and sectors as exceptions to the rule. They are framed as people and companies doing something that they're not meant to, as opposed to exactly what all the economic orthodoxies demand they do.

The more difficult truth is that the economic status quo not only accepts businesses that harm our health – it incentivises and demands they do so. Profit at the expense, and through the exploitation of, health is a ubiquitous part of current economic and corporate orthodoxies. As such, any critique of individual businesses which is not couched in the terms of political economy or critique of our economic orthodoxy constitutes – mostly unintentionally – to a dangerous obfuscation of this fact. It communicates the idea that a minority are ruining it for the majority, rather than the reality that the orthodoxy is broken, or that the rules of the game are stacked against the health of the many.

There's no single figure on how much national or global profit rests on health exploitation. But a thought experiment suggests it happens at an immense scale. If we were to imagine an index of all the corporations who profit in some way from poor health, it would certainly include the obvious candidates: tobacco, alcohol, sugary drinks, fast food, confectionery and gambling products. It would also include companies at the heart of climate change, whether fossil fuel companies, or those with large carbon footprints. It would include social media companies, for their impact on mental health. It could cover fashion, beauty and cosmetics sectors, for the same reason. It would cover a whole host of companies with poor records on occupational health and workplace equality – gig economy leaders (Deliveroo, Uber), those with famously poor workplace standards (Sports Direct, Amazon), and those who undermine worker rights, through schemes like Fire and Rehire (from British Gas to Weetabix). It would also include companies that inflict long working hours, stress, or unequal pay on their workforce; those in advertising and product design and those who provide help to any of the above with their strategy, promotions, or branding.

In short, it would cover nearly every major corporation going. There are very few businesses whose profits do not come with some net health cost to the population, albeit of varying scale. This suggests we need campaigns and policies that look beyond the individual bad practice of the worst offenders. Instead, we need to look at the dynamics of the exploitative relationship between capital and health.

This is a challenging fact for the nature of our public health campaigns. Our most visible and best funded public health campaigns are almost always quite targeted. Recent examples include minimum unit pricing of alcohol, increased taxes on tobacco, plain packaging of cigarettes, limits on fixed odds betting terminals, a crackdown on 'loot boxes' in online games or a crackdown on adverts for junk food to children on TV and online. It is very hard to find a public health campaign that anchors itself around a macro-critique of the economic orthodoxy, rather than a micro-critique of the practices of a small number of businesses or an individual sector.

There are some instances where ideas and slogans have suggested a broader focus, particularly in distinctly left campaigns. But closer inspection often exposes superficiality. 'People before profit' is one good example that often appears in the health sector.[23] The words suggest a broad critique of our economic model, and its enablement of poor health.

But, when used in the health context – even in the diversity of its use by a range of public health and radical campaign groups – this idea is almost always targeted at individual sectors and business practices: most often the pharmaceutical, health insurance or direct health provider businesses.[24] In its narrow focus, it fails to provide a genuine, conceptual challenge to the economic orthodoxy. We can trace through some specific examples of this in practice.

In the US, Bernie Sanders has been one of the longest standing proponents of 'people before profit'. In his final debate with Joe Biden during the 2020 Democratic Primaries, he argued:

> If you want to guarantee quality health care to all, not make $100 billion in profit for the health care industry, you know what you need? . . . You need to take on the drug companies and the insurance companies.

Here, as elsewhere, Sanders makes clear that people before profit is a critique of two or three sectors – not a full critique of health's position with our economic model.

Similar examples can be found in UK politics and campaigns, as well. In the months before the 2019 general election, the Labour Party released the policy document *Medicines for the Many: Public Health before Private Profit*.[25] The document focused, almost exclusively on one sector: pharmaceutical companies. It outlined a comprehensive plan to bring more public control over R&D, drug prices and medicine manufacture. That is, it was another example of the language of broad economic critique being betrayed by a narrow focus on one sector.

Problematically, the sectors chosen as the focal point of the left's critique are almost always those explicitly within 'healthcare'. This is another example of the NHS forming the single horizon of how big and bold we're currently willing to be when it comes to radical health.

This chapter is not an apologia for individual businesses or sectors that find themselves held to account or shamed because they make a negative contribution to the sum of the nation's health. Rather, it's an argument that very targeted micro-economic critiques of individual businesses and sectors are simply not radical enough to generate the level of progress we need, and which is possible. At best, such critiques constitute incrementalism.

While the pursuit of small gains is a sometimes sound strategy, the last 100 years should have provided proof that major victories for health – at least, victories that would go against the interests of capital – rarely emerge from an incremental approach of targeting the worst corporate offenders 'one at a time'. I've already highlighted our difficulties in putting the tobacco industry to bed. Even more alarming is the emergence of equivalent public health threats – i.e., those that cause epidemic level health consequences, which market their products aggressively and which use 'tobacco tactics' to lobby against public health measures – in other categories.

Big food and drink are behind a doubling in global adult obesity and at least a quintupling of childhood obesity in the UK since the 1980s.[26] Alcohol and opioids are tangibly slowing life expectancy in the USA.[27] Study after study shows gambling addiction figures may be far worse than thought, with ever more severe mental health impacts being recorded in recent research.[28]

We need to break out from our current game of 'public health whack-a-mole' – where, as one threat is suppressed (very slowly, and with huge collective effort), a new one emerges. We can only bypass this with a more fundamental critique, and with broader, more ambitious and more conceptual policy. This is the opportunity offered by the economic frontier.

HEALTH AND CAPITAL: THE BEVERIDGE REPORT

Moving from a 'micro' (individual businesses) to 'macro' (whole economy) critique means understanding the fundamentals of the relationship between our health and capital. The nature of this relationship defines the value placed on good health, the level of intervention the state is willing to consider to protect health and whether health exploitation by capital is normalised, or even actively encouraged.

The terms of this relationship aren't static. Rather, they evolve and change over time. Exploring these shifts can help us understand how the value of health is bound by political and economic norms. As the origin of modern welfare, the 'Beveridge report' provides perhaps the best place to begin.

William Beveridge's best-selling policy report *Social Security and Allied Services* (1942) defined the design of the British welfare state, including through the recommendation of the formation of a health service. It is sometimes noted that William Beveridge was an unlikely founding father for such a significant expansion in welfare. For a short time a Liberal MP,[29] then a Liberal peer, Beveridge was not always a man with whom state intervention sat easy. While the report for which he is almost exclusively now known was highly interventionist, Beveridge went through long periods of fierce opposition to a large and active state. As Margaret Jones and Rodney Lowe note in their book on British welfare, Beveridge was even uncomfortable with the very word 'welfare':

> Even the supposed founder of the welfare state, Sir William Beveridge, disliked the 'Santa Claus' – or the 'something for nothing' – connotations of the term [welfare]. He preferred 'social service state', which emphasised not just social rights but also individual responsibilities.[30]

Any reluctance Beveridge had was eased by what he believed welfare – including health provision – could offer the market-based economy. Beveridge saw a state-backed health offer as integral to building a thriving and productive economy following the massive destruction of the Second World War.

> The first principle is that any proposals for the future, while they should use to the full the experience gathered in the past, should not be restricted by consideration of sectional interests established in the obtaining of that experience. Now, when the war is abolishing landmarks of every kind, is the opportunity for using experience in a clear field. A revolutionary moment in the world's history is a time for revolutions, not for patching.
>
> [. . .]
>
> The third principle is that social security must be achieved by co-operation between the State and the individual. The State should offer security for service and contribution. The state in organising security should not stifle incentive, opportunity, responsibility; in establishing a national minimum, it should leave room and encouragement for voluntary action by each individual to provide more than that minimum for himself and his family.[31]

The final paragraph is telling. The idea of 'security for service and contribution' suggests a welfare system predicated on supporting to the extent workers can do their duty within markets – and indeed, conditional upon it. The idea of a national minimum, with room for *every* family to provide more than that, suggests a preoccupation with incentives and competition integral to the running of markets. Health and welfare for

Beveridge were valuable for what they could provide in terms of market sustenance and productivity.

Put another way, health was a *means to an end* in the Beveridge report – where the end was thriving markets and productive employment.

A treatment-orientated National Health Service[32] has proven to be an ideal intervention if the objective is to support markets with increased human capital. As an acute service, it does not constrain markets, or force them to consider health as part of some sense of social purpose. It does provide them with a boost, in the form of a healthier workforce ('human capital'). As an intervention, it has helped deliver huge health improvements – but improvements that have plateaued at the point the average person can expect to maintain 'reasonable health' until almost exactly the age of retirement, and to live in below reasonable health thereafter.[33] That is, the length of the average healthy life has now plateaued at the age 'service and contribution' – normally – end.

HEALTH AND CAPITAL: THE AUSTERITY DECADE

This political relationship between health and wealth has evolved from the relationship prescribed by William Beveridge in the 1940s. If health is a means to an end in the Beveridge Report, there has been a fundamental reversal today. The norm in 2020s Britain is not that good health is the basis for a good economy – but that output growth is the fundamental basis, and condition, for good health.

At the turn of the 2010 decade, there was rhetoric suggesting that concepts like health, wellbeing and quality of life would be prioritised over overly blunt considerations like growth. On 25 November 2010, David Cameron gave a major speech on wellbeing:

> But I do think it's high time we admitted that, taken on its own, GDP is an incomplete way of measuring a country's progress. Of course, it shows you that the economy is growing, but it doesn't show you how that growth is created . . . Let me give you some domestic examples, if you like, of this issue . . . We've had something of a cheap booze free-for all – again, supposed to be good for growth, but were we really thinking about the impact of that on law and order and on wellbeing? We've had something of an irresponsible media and marketing free-for-all – again, this was meant to be good for growth, but what about the impact on childhood? It's because of this fundamentally flawed

approach that for decades Western societies have seen the line of GDP rising steadily upwards, but at the same time, levels of contentment have remained static or have even fallen.[34]

In some very isolated instances, there was some policy consistent with this fleeting embrace of wellbeing. Putting cigarettes behind screens was implemented in shops and supermarkets, despite being unpopular with right wing think tanks and the big tobacco corporate lobby. Less successful were short-lived plans for a 'Pasty Tax', which became one of George Osborne's more embarrassing U-turns.

Overall, the policy impact was marginal at best. The associated data, the ONS' national measure of well-being is flimsy, rarely cited and has little to no bearing on decisions. In retrospect, the wellbeing rhetoric did little more than provide a convenient distraction from the fact that austerity represented a fundamental reinforcement of growth as our predominant goal, and GDP as our dominant metric.

With hindsight, David Cameron's focus served as little more than a distraction, for the public and media, from an obsessive preoccupation with output growth. His first speech as premier was titled 'Transforming the British economy: Coalition strategy for economic growth' and mentioned the word 17 times further.[35] Growth was made synonymous with recovery. The plank that linked growth with austerity for the Cameron regime was the idea that public spending either inflates debt or increases taxes, suppressing growth. It is a logic that suggests public spending cuts are necessary to support prosperity.

The idea was enacted with relish. Between 2010/11 and 2014/15, the Department of Communities and Local Government (now the Ministry of Housing, Communities and Local Government) saw a real change in its budget of around minus 50 per cent. The Department of Work and Pensions saw a reduction of 30 per cent. Almost as hard hit were the Departments of Justice; Culture, Media and Sport; Environment, Food and Rural Affairs; as well as the Home Office.[36] The NHS was subjected to one of the greatest funding squeezes in its history, leading it to the brink of collapse by the end of the decade.

The point is this. Austerity's starting point was that growth in output measures, like GDP, should be the ultimate goal of policy and the economy. It also proposed that cuts to public spending were crucial both to maximising growth and ensuring that growth was sustainable (a view, needless to say, that has been entirely discredited since).[37] That means that, according to austerity, cutting health and wellbeing budgets were the best way to improve national health and wellbeing.

In 1948, Beveridge saw health investment as critical to sustaining the market-based economy after a major crisis: a means to an end. In the 2010s, austerity positioned health investment as a deflator on prosperity. Our health was framed as a *luxury* product – one that could rarely be afforded and, even when it could, was unlikely to be the optimal place to put our money. Put another way, the 1940s notion that our prosperity is conditional on our good health transformed to one that suggested good health is conditional on growth in economic output.

ALIGNMENT WITH ECONOMIC ORTHODOXY

In many ways, the transformed positionality of health from Beveridge to Cameron reflects a change in the economic orthodoxies since the 1940s and the 2010s. It is consistent with the transition from a broadly Keynesian to a broadly neoliberal economic consensus.

In her book *Doughnut Economics*, Kate Raworth documents how modern economics became obsessed with growth.[38] From the creation of the 'Gross National Value' measure by Simon Kuznets in the 1930s, she traces how traditional economic models have developed to support the idea that growth in GDP is the objective goal. A range of organisations have emerged to support, embed and normalise the idea (the OECD, Bretton Woods) – and the kinds of simplified, imperfect models and graphs that dominate orthodox school and university economic textbooks work to much the same effect. The right's ability to create a political reality where health is conditional on GDP further supports this transition, and reiterates the idea of GDP as a sole goal of society and the economy. In turn, it supports and strengthens the grip of a neoliberal political economy.

Raworth also points out that we haven't always made prosperity and growth synonymous. Twenty-first century economists have a choice about the world they want to create, and that doesn't have to be one organised exclusively around output growth. In her words: 'For over half a century, economists have fixated on GDP as the first measure of economic progress, but GDP is a false God waiting to be ousted.'[39] That is, we have a choice about whether we want to accept health's subordination to GDP.

When considering about this, we should begin from the realisation that output growth measures like GDP are very poor metrics. In a speech to students in Kansas, John F. Kennedy famously critiqued the limitations of such measures:

> Our Gross National Product, now, is over $800 billion dollars a year . . . but the gross national product does not allow for the health of our children, the quality of their education or the joy of their play. It does not include the beauty of our poetry or the strength of our marriages, the intelligence of our public debate or the integrity of our public officials. It measures neither our wit nor our courage, neither our wisdom nor our learning, neither our compassion nor our devotion to our country, it measures everything in short, except that which makes life worthwhile.[40]

Decades later, and the climate movement has created a full body of evidence showing how GDP is not conductive to other societal goals, such as tackling the climate emergency itself.[41] The same is true of health. In Autumn last year, I worked with analysts at Lane Clark & Peacock (LCP) to examine what explained health improvement, and the big health inequalities that exist between regions in England. The biggest correlates were poverty, wealth inequality, income inequality, childhood education and access to sustainable healthy diets. GDP, by contrast, was an almost entirely useless predictor.

There are then two problems with the view the health should be conditional on output growth (rather than vice versa). First, growth alone does not predict better or more just health outcomes, meaning health won't just improve with GDP improvements. And second, because GDP is such a poor measure of health, policies introduced from the perspective of improving output growth are highly unlikely to be the same policies that would best support health and wellbeing.

In fact, that GDP is a poor measure of good health is only half the problem with the status quo. Equally troubling is the fact that GDP actively values both illness and the activities that generate poor health.[42]

First, it measures the economic activities that make us sick in the first place. Despite the fact that childhood obesity has risen from under 2 per cent in the 1980s (5–10 years olds) to 10 per cent in reception and 21 per cent in year 6 in 2020, junk food production and sales still make a full contribution to GDP.[43] Despite the fact that alcohol-related deaths reached record levels in 2020, the alcohol market still makes a full, unweighted contribution to GDP.[44] Despite the fact problem or addiction gambling has reached more than 2 million in the UK, gambling is still counted uncritically within GDP.[45]

This ill health is then counted a second time. In the most recent accounts, approximately 5 per cent of the UK's GDP was linked to healthcare expenditure.[46] This means the volume of treatments, diagnostics and other operations all contribute to GDP figures. If an unhealthy product puts us in hospital, that's double bubble as far as GDP is concerned. But if regulation justified on someone out of hospital by reducing consumption, GDP feels the cost two-fold – in the reduced business activity, and in the reduction in avoidable acute healthcare treatments and services.[47]

So the status quo relationship between health and the economy perpetuates three things. First, it (wrongly) implies that growth is the best way to improve health, supporting the orthodox dominance of GDP (and similar measures). Second, and in turn, it thereby props up measures that do not value health and actively value poor health (both the economic practices that cause poor health, and the resulting hospital activity). Thirdly, it incentivises a health model where a) very little is done to encourage corporations to create good health and b) very little is done to support good health before a diagnosis, in line with the principles of Chapter Two.

The cost of this entirely sub-optimal approach to health falls not on the wealthy, nor on the corporations who profit from poor health, Rather, it falls on taxpayers and the state. The former chief executive of the NHS in England – Lord Simon Stevens – put it well in 2015:

> Because we have a tax-funded National Health Service in this country, rather than employer-based health insurance like the French or Germans or Americans, we don't saddle business with the costs of health care.[48]

If companies make us sick, we pick up the bill – collectively as taxpayers. Executives and shareholders only reap the profits. And that means, at least to some extent, our proud system of publicly funded and universal healthcare has been transformed into a subsidy on those who exploit our health for profit.

Moreover, the costs of poor health are extensive. Recent modelling shows that obesity – among just the current cohort of children – will cost almost half a trillion to the NHS and wider society, over the course of their lives. Childhood mental health will cost £120 billion per year by 2040.[49]

If we don't change this reality, everything else in the rest of this book becomes much harder to deliver. Each chapter, except this one, outlines steps towards a state intervention for radically improving our health. Yet, if those simply subsidise poor business behaviours – or worse, create space for or incentivise new sites and types of exploitation – their impact will be limited, and the political appetite for radical change reduced.

A recalibration of the health/wealth relationship isn't just important in its own terms, it is integral for the integrity of the vision put forward in this book more widely.

NOT A BINARY CHOICE

We needn't see this as a choice between Beveridge's and our modern conception of the health/capital relationship. That would be a false dichotomy. Though Beveridge's conception is evidently preferrable, it has its own limitations.

Beveridge's conception of the relationship between health and economy can be critiqued from a few different perspectives. Feminist critiques of the Beveridge report are particularly well known.[50] In looking to maintain the economic status quo, the interventions prescribed by Beveridge were often a reflection of the patriarchal norms of the 1940s. In ignoring gender as a unit of analysis, his work and the policy it influenced allowed existing and repressive power relations to be reiterated. Alarmingly, Beveridge's report actively distinguishes between men and women – and makes its proposals explicitly dependent on the idea that women will contribute disproportionately to welfare, by providing unpaid labour, social reproduction and care.

For Beveridge, the role of the state and the married woman was to enable the productive, economically active and employed working-age man. That this was the dominant consideration in the origin and structure of welfare, and by implication the NHS, continues to have a bearing on healthcare today. This is reflected in the rates of misdiagnosis of endometriosis, and well documented reports of women being told their symptoms are trivial. It is reflected in how the 'hysterical woman' archetype has underpinned a reluctance to provide pain relief for women having coil fittings. It is epitomised by the exclusion of women from historic medical research on the basis that their hormones might impact the science.

There are equally strong critiques of the Beveridge report's focus on productivity by disabled rights campaigners.[51] Beveridge's schemes, which assume the role of welfare is to get people into work, anchor the kinds of discourse which split the country into 'scroungers' and 'shirkers' – a dynamic taken up and politically exploited by the Cameron/Osborne axis. The focus on productivity gives little scope to unconditionally valuing social justice, nor does it consider how discrimination, or a lack of tailored support, might make it harder for disabled people to access work – beyond the one-size-fits-all welfare package prescribed.

The explicit focus on productivity within the welfare state, as well as the inattention played to power dynamics by Beveridge, means services were and remain primarily designed around the needs of working age, able-bodied white men.

Critiques of Beveridge withstanding, we can still quantify the cost of a move from the kind of system he implemented, to a more brutal and small state version during austerity. This cost can be put in both economic and human terms. The redefinition of public spending on public health as unhealthy saw the UK's ability to prevent good health stall. This departure from our previous trajectory has cost over 130,000 lives, by best estimates.[52] Other research shows economic harm. In early 2018, a team led by Professor Clare Bambra found that a third of the productivity gap between the North of England and the rest of England was explained by disparities in health. They concluded that closing this gap would add £13.2 billion to the economy in just the first year.[53] My estimates in 2020 suggest the economic value of closing this disparity has risen further: to £20 billion.[54] That's approximately twice the gross value added to the economy by the whole of UK agriculture.[55]

We need not be bound to models that came before. The potential for transformative change is for improvements beyond merely readopting a Beveridge model. The specific opportunity is to go beyond the view of health as only valuable insofar as it is good for capital and markets, or the view that it is a luxury good that cannot be afforded because it suppresses capital and markets, to instead view health as a key societal objective and measure – an end in and of itself.

PROTECTING HEALTH FOR THE MANY

Understanding the role it plays within current economic orthodoxy opens up huge opportunities for improving our health. In particular, there are three breaks from the past we can and should look to make:

- We need to allocate health a value in its own right, in contrast to both the Beveridge and Cameron conceptions, which subordinate it to suspect economic orthodoxies.
- We need a target that captures the value of good health and poor health, in a way GDP does not.
- We need a system to transfer liability for poor health created by capital, onto capital itself.

Based on these criteria, there is a strong case for a new target that values health in its own right, and takes aim at the current scope for health exploitation. We might call this a **Public Health Net Zero** (PHN-ZERO) target. Broadly conceived, PHN-ZERO targets a state where it is no longer possible to profit from poor health – an enactment of 'people before profit', for the whole economy.

PHN-ZERO provides an immediate decision point – should we endorse highly interventionist government policy and regulation, or give businesses the chance to set voluntary targets and Corporate Social Responsibility (CSR) schemes? It is important to be clear from the outset that CSR rarely sustains the radical changes needed to properly protect our health. PHN-ZERO cannot be left to shareholder whims or voluntary targets.

Sometimes, voluntary schemes simply do nothing. In the last few years, Public Health England have overseen a 'challenge' from government to the food and drink industry – to remove 20 per cent of the sugar from foods that contribute most to children's sugar consumption. The hope was that the market and the sector could solve the problem themselves, without any need for state intervention. However, since the challenge began in 2016, they have managed to remove just 3 per cent of sugar.[56] It has been little more than a distraction.

In other cases, CSR schemes have provided yet another tool for health exploitation. A 2020 paper led by Mark Petticrew found corporate social responsibility materials from the alcohol industry were chock-a-block with 'dark nudges' – behavioural queues which are designed to encourage people to take actions not in their self-interest – which acted to normalise and encourage drinking.[57] For example, the first sentence of an industry CSR leaflet about the link between alcohol and cancer:[58] 'There is no scientific consensus on why some people develop cancer and some don't'.[59] This sows needless uncertainty: there is strong consensus among the scientific community that differential alcohol use is one reason some people develop cancer, and some do not.[60]

The target of a PHN-ZERO would need to be actively delivered through state intervention, and actively managed by government – specifically, by a new, empowered arm or office within government, with extensive public health powers. I suggest a Government Public Health Unit, located in the Treasury – and with a Cabinet Level Minister, who should report on progress and new policy on an annual basis (as per the Chancellor). The rest of this chapter outlines three effective, evidenced and proportionate powers this unit should have in pursuing a PHN-ZERO, and in ensuring our health is valued in its own right and protected from the worse instincts of capital (*Table 3.1*).

Table 3.1   Proposed Powers for a New Government Public Health Unit

Power	Strategy
Fiscal Disincentive	Primary aim, to encourage changes in corporate behaviour; secondary aim, to raise revenue that subsidises direct public health intervention by the state
Regulation	Create liability for actions in areas and markets where tax is unlikely to be an effective mechanism to change business behaviours
Forms of Ownership	For stubborn problems and emerging threats, the ability to introduce new public-health focused ownership models – including state monopoly and common ownership.

Having talked to many, I am of the strong opinion that these proposed powers would be welcomed by most businesses. While a small number stand to lose out, and their lobbyists will make as much noise as they can, most businesses tell me they want a healthier country. They realise they stand to gain from better health. But they don't think they can achieve the scale of change needed on their own. Privately, they want bold government intervention to be enacted, and to create a level playing field.

This is exactly what PHN-ZERO would achieve: a healthier, fairer and more just economic model, that works for the many.

Fiscal Disincentives

The first strand of delivering a policy like PHN-ZERO is shifting the cost of health exploitation from individuals to capital. Fiscal disincentives have proven effective in every instance they've been used to support public health. One excellent case study is the Soft Drinks Industry Levy (SDIL).

Introduced in the 2016 budget, it added a charge of 24 pence/L on drinks containing 8 grams of sugar per 100ml and 18 pence/L on those with between 5 grams and 8 grams of sugar per 100ml.[61] As such, the first benefit of the sugary drinks industry levy was revenue generation. According to official government figures, the levy raised £240 million in 2018 to 2019. Revenue went up in the year 2019 to 2020, to £336 million.[62] That is money that can be invested in health. At the time of writing, the Treasury is still due to announce what it plans to do with what is now £760 millions of income – having committed that every penny will be invested in improving the health of children.[63]

Even more impressively, the levy has led to a significant reduction in the amount of sugar in drinks themselves. The brilliance of public health taxes, particularly those that are designed with thresholds as in the case of the SDIL, is that companies are often very reluctant to either absorb the cost (from profits) or pass it to the consumer (in price). In reaction, the vast majority decided it was in their interest to make their product healthier themselves. The average drink captured by the levy has gone on to reduce its sugar content by 43.7 per cent.[64] They did so in the knowledge that choosing to do otherwise would leave them incredibly vulnerable to new, healthier products entering the market – with lower costs.

The third benefit is remarkable, given the prophecies of doom woven by corporate lobbyists between the levy being announced and implemented. It is this: health taxes did not harm businesses. An analysis of stock market returns from soft drinks companies showed that they'd actually experienced long-run growth following the tax.[65] That is, the state pushing them to become healthier improved their business model

– by making them more sustainable, by enforcing innovation, or otherwise raising their profile.

It might come as a surprise that an initiative pioneered under David Cameron's first majority government – and which austerity chancellor George Osborne has named one of his proudest policies – is the first cited in this section. It is of course important to recognise that a sugary drinks industry levy alone is not immune from many of the problems discussed in this chapter – in particular, it is too specific in its aims to change the basis of the relationship between health and capital.

Conservative governments have since shown that this policy is an exception, rather than the rule. In July 2021 a government-commissioned independent report was published entitled *The National Food Strategy*, which recommended scaling up unhealthy food levies to raise £3 billion. With a backdrop of consternation from the ranks of the Conservative Party, the proposal was dismissed out of hand by ministers. Elsewhere, public health policy both before and during Covid has shown how ideologically uncomfortable the right are with the implications of putting public health first – and shifting the onus for health away from the individual onto corporations.

The true test of PHN-ZERO is not whether there are one-off good examples of public health-led fiscal policies – implemented to keep public health campaigners satiated and distracted from more systemic problems. The test is whether it can be targeted towards a more fundamental shift in our economy, to entirely and evenly shift the cost of health exploitation away from individuals and onto capital.

There are a range of places where we can follow sound international examples in fundamentally increasing our ambition. Continuing with the theme of food and drink, for example, the UK could follow Mexico and Hungary's example, and expand the levy on sugary drinks to all unhealthy food and drink. Hungary's version of this tax dates back to 2011, and covers all pre-packaged products with added sugar, chocolates, salted snacks and energy drinks. In just three years, as many as 73 per cent of consumers had reduced consumption of these products – even though most of this tax wasn't reflected in increased prices.[66] Mexico's tax goes further still and covers all foods with greater calorific density than 275kcal/100g. Evaluations again show that diets have improved since the policy was introduced.[67]

PHN-ZERO does not need to be limited to unhealthy goods, like junk food and alcohol. As the previous chapter indicated, there are many business activities that generate poor health outcomes – from renting out homes that aren't fit for purpose, to reneging on occupational health standards, or allowing discrimination and inequality to thrive in the workplace. These are all health-negative activities amenable to fiscal disincentives. Like the Sugary Drinks Industry Levy, their ambition would primarily be disincentivising corporate exploitation and changing business behaviour – with revenue creation a secondary aim.

For example, new fiscal interventions on causes of poor health in the workplace could give much needed teeth to some of the reporting targets recently brought in on equality standards, particularly regarding the gender pay gap. Despite new legislation brought in under the Theresa May government, which required companies over a certain size to report on pay disparities, unfair pay has remained prevalent. In 2020, the median gender pay gap sat at 16 per cent.[68] An investigation the year before had shown that, despite reporting requirements, four in ten big businesses were reporting a widening gender pay gap.[69]

The pay gap is commonly described as a case of economic injustice, but less often as a health injustice. Yet, the discrepancy (and the discrimination that unpins it) does come with tangible impacts on both women's physical and mental health. One study, carried out in America, showed that women paid less for equal work were more likely to experience depression and anxiety, amongst other mental health consequences.[70]

Pay inequality has a snowball effect. According to the Office for National Statistics, British women will earn £263,000 less than their male counterparts over their life.[71] The consequences of this significant discrepancy in wealth accumulation are likely to be particularly pronounced in later life, when a lower salary and smaller pension constitute twin problems. According to the Chartered Institute of Insurance, a woman can expect to have pension wealth worth £35,700 by the time she reaches 65–69. This is a fifth of the average amongst men the same age.[72] This economic vulnerability can lead to a host of socially undesirable and avoidable outcomes – including worse outcomes for longevity and health-state life expectancy.

There is no reason a levy design could not scale the design of existing public health levies. Based on the conception that both health improvement and health justice rely on equal pay, staggered penalties could simply be linked to the final pay gap announced by companies – based on total employee pay. In all likelihood, it would only take a small penalty to drive forward significant change – and given pay gaps tend to be linked to other drivers of occupational injustice, it is almost certain that public health improvements would be observed.

These are just examples of where a large tax-led 'pay or play' approach could begin. In many ways, the specific examples I've given are far less important than the concept – there is huge opportunity for public health taxes to raise money, improve health and create a more sustainable relationship between health and capital.

Regulation

While an expansive regime of financial disincentives is essential to the PHN-ZERO agenda, it is not the complete answer. There are cases where fiscal disincentives will be less effective, or simply more difficult to implement. In these cases, there is an opportunity for the creative use of expanded regulation.

Public health regulation can be both highly effective and incredibly popular. Take for instance the ban on smoking in enclosed public places and workplaces, introduced in 2007. The policy has been effective on its own terms by contributing to lower smoking rates. Just one year after the ban, research in the *British Medical Journal* estimated that there had been 1,200 fewer hospital admissions for heart attacks – with the British Heart Foundation attributing the legislation to this success.[73] But this measure is perhaps most interesting because of its rise in popularity after implementation. Many will remember the fierce debate around the right to smoke indoors, often framed around civil liberty, the economy and the sustainability of pubs. Today, debate has turned into consensus, as 83 per cent now support the ban – including 52 per cent of smokers.[74]

One area where fiscal disincentive may work less well, and this kind of regulation could contribute, is in the digital economy. Digital taxes have proven difficult to administer. First, because tax is paid from the base of manufacture rather than at the point of delivery, allowing digital giants to plant their HQ somewhere with low tax rates ('profit shifting').[75] Digital business models don't comply with national boundaries in the way normal 'brick and mortar' businesses do. Second, digital regulation often relies on international consensus – which proves difficult to arrive at, given certain nation-state's vested interests in maintaining the current status quo (particularly America's). Third, a lack of transparency over profits makes it hard to target and enforce specific taxes on unhealthy practices – a key design element for public health levies. Fourth, the make-up of the digital economy makes it hard to design taxes that genuinely change corporate behaviour, limiting its advantages. And finally, many of the harms that are caused by social media come from activities that are too toxic to be used for income generation (illegal activities such as grooming or harassment, for example).

For PHN-ZERO to be viable, it needs to have the ability to react to these kinds of challenges.

The digital economy is a sophisticated system of health exploitation. On the one hand, there is an element of dependency. Equal outcomes among children depend on digital access – with Covid-19 and school closures exposing the injustice faced by the one million children and families without adequate access to a device or connectivity in their home.[76] But the digital divide is not the only important measure. The ability to safely access a wide variety of platforms – including social media – is vital in terms of ensuring children have access to the networks, digital literacy and other skills they will inevitably need in the future.[77] Indeed, I have already put forward digital as a key component in a Universal Public Health Service (Chapter Two).

This means bans and content filters are unlikely to be adequate solutions. If all children find their digital and social media use restricted, it will leave them playing catch-up in their adult life.[78] And if our solution to inequality is to restrict digital access to the most disadvantaged children, we will exclude them from the skills, social interactions and networks that will define their future outcomes.

Nonetheless, we cannot ignore the public health risks. Cyberbullying and online harassment affect almost one in ten children aged 10 to 15 in England and can introduce severely negative psychosocial outcomes for victims – including depression and anxiety.[79] Social media has also been linked to social isolation, peer pressure and exposure to inaccurate, unsuitable, or dangerous content.[80] Ofcom, the communications regulator, has shown that eight in ten children between the ages of 12 and 15 have at least one harmful online experience a year – in most cases, relating to interactions with other people or interactions with inappropriate content. For 4 per cent, this was material showing child sexual abuse. For 6 per cent, material encouraging terrorism. For 10 per cent, it was cyberstalking; for another 10 per cent pressure to send photos to another person; and for 15 per cent, it was violent or disturbing content.[81]

Often, the very activities that undermine the health and security of children (and adults) prove highly profitable for social media companies.

In some cases, the link between profit motive and harm can be focused on something ubiquitous. For example, a major method of monetising social media platforms is advertising revenue. Those advertisements are often used, intentionally, to expose children to harmful products, or content that would be more explicitly regulated on television. In 2017, I developed two major surveys – the Youth Obesity Policy Survey and the Youth Alcohol Policy Survey – as part of one of the biggest studies of children and young people ever carried out in the UK. A body of analysis emerging from these surveys shows, beyond doubt, that big food and drink and big alcohol companies are using social media platforms to target kids.[82]

There is also profit to be found in less prevalent, but higher harm content. Social media companies exist in ad supported ecosystems. These systems have not been designed to distinguish between harmful and harmless, legal and illegal content. So, when a gunman killed 49 people at two New Zealand mosques in 2019, and live streamed the incident, Facebook drew an audience and made a profit. When children are exposed to sexual material, or return to conversations with someone grooming them, they generate a profit for the platform.

Regulation can enact the spirit of fiscal disincentives. Public health taxes work on a 'play or pay' basis. They do not force corporations to focus on our health. But they enact sufficient incentive that a) it becomes far less profitable not to do so and b) people impacted have the means, through the state, to exact a price for poor health. In this case, legal accountability can enact this principle. For example, a new regulator with sweeping powers could transform social media, by making certain harms criminal, and introducing civil liability for others. Crucially, this should not be limited to a narrow definition, but should extend the full range of opportunities for the health exploitation from which social media companies currently profit.

Regulation could then be based on a transparent duty of care. A basis for this could be the approach taken in Canada to alcohol, where establishments serving drinks have a 'duty of care' to their patrons. This is a law that ensures commercial liability when harm emerges after drinking in a licenced establishment. In 2017, a British Colombia court found a pub 25 per cent liable when a drunk-driving accident left a pedestrian with a brain injury.[83]

The duty of care in Canada works as follows: you owe a duty to patrons not to overserve. If this happens, they are owed a duty – to be kept safe.

The same duty extended to social media would mean people within the commercial environment – i.e., on a social media site – would be owed safety. Standards of safety could be adopted from a range of other countries. In Germany, the NetzDG law (2018) demands all companies with more than two million registered users set up firm procedures to review content complaints with 24 hours.[84] In the European Union, there is a one hour time limit to take down extremist content.

Where that Duty of Care is not maintained, then liability should come into play. This could include the German approach of massive fines or, better still, the approach taken in Australia – where the *Sharing of Abhorrent Violent Material Act* (2019) introduced criminal penalties for social media executives and fines worth up to 10% of global turnover.

Vitally, any scheme must include full compensation for the person impacted (as opposed to the government alone). This would help encourage people to report harmful materials, and ensure the linkage of those that experience health consequences and those who benefit from health reparations.

Ownership Models

Finally, there is a strong case for using ownership models in the pursuit of a Public Health Net Zero. Ownership models and public control are less frequently discussed in the context of public health. However, they are well evidenced, impactful and revenue creating.

There is a particularly strong case for moving away from private ownership models in the case of fiscal/regulatory interventions which aren't working ('stubborn challenges') – or in the case of new products of public health concern ('new threats'). The specific ownership models used could themselves be varied. We could employ public ownership in some cases – with the Public Health Net Zero Unit empowered to bring distribution into direct public control. Equally, it could see the state enact the conditions for common ownership, to ensure certain resources are only used for purposes with a clear societal benefit.

Direct state control of distribution has been incredibly successful in reducing harm in countries that have used it – most commonly, for the distribution of alcohol.[85] In Sweden, the Swedish Alcohol Retailing Monopoly has the sole right to retail alcoholic beverages. Its website declares 'the purpose is to minimize alcohol related problems by selling alcohol in a responsible way, without profit motive'.[86] There are 400 stores and 500 sales agendas, and the country is free from aggressive alcohol advertising.[87] Similar systems can be found in all Nordic countries except Denmark, and in all Canadian provinces except Alberta.

Direct public ownership of a long-standing and hard to control public health threat has proved remarkably successful. A 2017 study found that if Sweden were to privatise its alcohol retail monopoly, alcohol consumption would increase by as much as 31 per cent. All else remaining the same, that increase in alcohol consumption would be expected to increase alcohol-related deaths by 42 per cent and assaults by 34 per cent.[88] As with other public health measures, while people are sometimes suspicous of their impact before they are implemented, large levels of public support and trust generally then follow. In Sweden, the system has 78 per cent support.[89]

In countries that choose state monopoly, the revenue opportunities are significant – and normally greater than from 'duties' on a private system (as in the UK). Because of the elimination of profit margins, and the vast array of tactics beyond price open to a state alcohol operator to control consumption, there are even examples of state monopolies keeping unit prices lower than private competitors *and* generating more revenue for the state.[90]

In the case of alcohol, state involvement tends to have occurred because it has proven a stubborn threat. Alcohol harms have long been clear in society and have proven less than amenable to other public health interventions. This has justified direct action to both maintain the availability of the product, and to achieve a state where its use is balanced – a sustainable relationship between civil liberty and public health. However, the experience of public ownership and state monopoly can provide a lesson in supporting the controlled introduction of new products that may otherwise have public health harms – a method of safely introducing things the market might not be trusted with.

For example, there is now a strong precedent across the world for the legalisation of cannabis. It was legalised in Canada for recreational purposes in 2018; in Georgia following a court ruling in 2018; in 17 US States, and in a host of other countries, provinces and territories. And there is a public health case for legalisation of cannabis, it its own right.[91] At present, criminalisation of drugs has little basis in evidence – and is rightly suspected to be little more than an instrument of targeted coercion and control by the state. A publicly controlled, managed and legal supply chain could reduce arrests, which are disproportionately of

Black people (and themselves a predictor of poor health outcomes, not least because of alarmingly poor standards of prison health).

State monopoly provides a proactive way to restrict the harms of cannabis – through mechanics like price control, limits on shop density and controlled opening hours. In 2019, one study examining the lessons of public health monopolies for the legalisation of cannabis concluded that 'for public health and welfare, public monopolization is generally a preferable option'.[92] Similar support for state monopoly can be found in the wider academic literature.[93]

Moreover, the experience of giving the market control of legalised cannabis in parts of America have shown that it simply funnels profits to the usual suspects – wealthy investors, private equity companies and big business. As Kojo Koram has put it: 'those who have suffered most under the War on Drugs are . . . excluded from the wealth that is being generated in its transition to a legal market'.[94] Just 1 per cent of cannabis dispensaries in the USA are owned by Black people. State control can help alleviate this question of equity.[95]

State monopoly is not the only form of ownership that might help address stubborn challenges and emerging threats. For example, in the case of reaching PHN-ZERO in the digital economy, common ownership might be an option alongside the regulatory proposals I discussed above.

The health harms of the digital economy cannot be entirely separated from its ownership model. A lack of clear ownership rights of personal data means we can be manipulated by digital giants – whether directly, or in passing on sophisticated insights that help personalise products and advertising. That is, without ownership of our data, we have little insight into how it's being used and little control over to what end. We can be influenced to buy unhealthy products through personalised advertisements, which are more convincing and subtler than anything we've ever faced. Our dopamine receptors can be gamed, to increase our screen time and create addiction dynamics in our social media use – good for owners and advertisers, but disastrous for our mental health. Essentially, without ownership of our data, we neither have knowledge of how our data is used, nor power over its purpose and impact.

There is, therefore, a public health case for taking back ownership of data – both to maintain standards and set conditions on the purposes to which it is put by profit-making entities. In this case, the most viable ownership model is not state ownership, but common ownership, through a digital commons. A digital commons positions the state as a steward, not an owner, of the digital economy. Recommendations made by former John McDonnell advisor James Meadway, the Royal Society and the British Academy have all identified the need for such strong stewardship by the state in managing data.[96]

The digital commons is most often proposed in opposition to the two other options for managing the data economy: more competition (e.g. by breaking up monopolies) and more state intervention (e.g. through regulators). The advantage of the commons is that it prioritises the new forms of communal ownership that have emerged in the digital age and helps avoid unnecessary de-aggregation of data – which is exponentially more valuable when compiled.

There is no better body for delivering this kind of curation and stewardship than one focused on public health. As a distinct natural resource, data has been described as the 'new oil' – on the basis that it does not have innate value but can be imbued with significant value in the process of extraction.[97] But perhaps a more accurate comparison of data is 'the new water' – a natural resource we cannot live without, and which has the potential to cause disease and other health consequences if imbued with impurities. A public health approach to the data commons would place a primary focus on preventing harm, ensuring that the full cost and benefit of data's potential is taken into account whenever and whereever it is used.

The power of innovative ownership models for products that we want to safely distribute has been relatively untapped in the UK. Their power to radically improve health should be an integral part of the power of any new public health body, both for raising revenue and for achieving public health gains.

A NOTE ON POWER

PHN-ZERO offers the opportunity to revolutionise health by moving towards a model of active public health stewardship – by the state, in the collective interest and as an expression of a collective will.

This does not come without a need for caution. Public health interventions have long been plagued by accusations of paternalism, today often expressed through the concept of the 'nanny state'. This framing defines punitive interventions as attempts to control people, particularly poor people, based on the moral ideals of the public health establishment.

It would be foolish to suggest there has never been an element of power and control to the work of the public health movement. In the eighteenth century, the temperance movement reacted to the 'gin craze' in Great Britain with moralising absolutism. The founder of the Methodist Church, John Wesley, made the issue entirely black and white when calling both the sale and purchase of alcohol evil. The national debate at that point in time was driven by a desire for order by the middle and upper classes, rather than by any genuine interest in population health.

Equally, there must be a concept that allows us to collectively act in the interest of population health. When it comes to economic justice, the left is rarely timid in the face of exploitation. We do not simply tolerate the harms caused by business models like Bright House and Wonga because of civil liberty and the right of all to purchase consumer goods. We act, because the relationship these companies establish between people and capital is exploitative.

That means we must not be blind where injustice might be a consequence. For example, I have focused on the case study of food and drink, as one where taxation works. But in many cases, unhealthy food is often cheaper than healthy food – and if food prices were to rise it could create real difficulties for people already living in poverty. The onus is for any move towards fiscal disincentives not to constitute a penalty or restriction aimed at people without enough money. It must always be combined with mobilisation of revenue in targeted interventions, like subsidies or the kind of services outlined in the Universal Public Health Service. Indeed, the PHN-ZERO and the Universal Public Health Service could have a wonderfully reciprocal relationship, linking revenue creation with need alleviation.

This is the foundation on which an interventionist approach such as PHN-ZERO is justified. It is acceptable insofar as it eschews moralising and focuses on demonstrable exploitative relationships between health and capital. It is not about bans or absolutism, nor etiquette, morals, or standards. It is about prescribing health a value and prescribing a cost when actors – whether intentionally, or because of the environment in which they are competing – profit from poor health. It is about having the instruments to defend the many.

4

The Social Care Frontier

To date, the damage caused by Covid-19 has been disproportionately concentrated on those who rely on social care support. Throughout the pandemic, care homes were one of the key sites of excess mortality, despite government proclamations of protective rings and emergency funds. The first wave of the pandemic saw 30,000 more deaths among care home residents in England than we would have expected, almost all inevitable.[1] People who relied on care in their homes were also at extra risk – with 3,000 'excess deaths' during the first wave – and found themselves subject to by far the most severe impacts from lockdowns and other restrictions.

Older people, adults living with disabilities and people with long-term health conditions alike were critically let down by pandemic policies and left to cope with significantly greater risk.

However, whilst things were inevitably exasperated by poor government decisions during 2020/1, we must be careful not to erase longer-standing structural problems with how care is organised. The reason our social care system struggles – before the pandemic, and during it – is down to its neoliberal foundations. It is the political economy of care which undercuts its sustainability.

NEOLIBERALISM AND CARE

The post-war Clement Attlee government was very clear about the founding principles behind their National Health Service. It was far less clear about what core principles would sit behind the social care system. At best, the 1948 National Assistance Act gave some sense of what was to be expected from local authorities:

[they will] provide residential accommodation for persons who by reason of age, infirmity or any other circumstances are in need of care and attention which is not otherwise available to them.[2]

It was here that social care was set on a very different path to the National Health Service.

The clause 'not otherwise available to them' is critical. The implication is that local authorities need only use their budgets to meet the care needs of the worst off, or the very most in-need – a conception that allows a) private sector dominance; b) means testing and fees and c) a system built around intervening on acute need as late as possible, rather than addressing emerging needs as early as possible. Each underpins a problem faced in social care today.

Local authorities did continue to directly provide most care in the years following the act.[3] Indeed, Harold Wilson's government expanded their role to make provision of domestic help mandatory, and to cover home adaptations for both older and disabled people. By contrast, the independent sector remained a small stump, delivering a very small fraction of care services. Nonetheless, the 1948 legislation still allowed for the registration and inspection of profitable care providers; allowed fee charging independent services to be commissioned; and accepted the concept of personal payment for care.

This was a crucial enabler for the radical social care reforms implemented by the Thatcher governments. In general, her governments were very conscious of the problems posed by an ageing population. The projected speed of population ageing promised to place a bigger strain on public services, increasing demand on the state and, in turn, increasing state expenditure.

Nowhere would state expenditure go up faster than long-term care services. So, when they looked to isolate areas where state expenditure could be reduced – including by moving more service provision into the private sector – long-term care was a clear candidate.

The strategy focused on mobilising older people's money (through means tests) into an independent market (created through pump priming with public funds).[4] The approach wasn't a guarded secret. Indeed, in a review of the community care system, Roy Griffiths wrote:[5]

> Many of the elderly have higher incomes and levels of savings than in the past . . . this growth of individually held resources could provide a contribution to meeting community care needs.[6]

In the same document, he outlined his central idea of local authorities as 'brokers' of care, not direct providers. He suggested they act as 'the designers, organisers and purchasers of non-health services, and not primarily as direct providers' – that is, he imagined the local authority becoming the equivalent of a travel agent for the package care deals offered up by big private providers.[7]

When it came to creating a market, state resources were the basis for growing and sustaining a dominant independent sector. For instance, between 1980 and 1990, there was an explosion in the use of Supplementary Payment benefit – a form of social security – to fund places in private care homes. The process worked as follows. Previously, local authorities assessed care needs, and then put in plans to meet them. But in the 1980s, a new scheme was formalised whereby people could bypass their local authority's assessment and use national welfare budgets to take an immediate place in an 'independent' sector care home. As Stewart Player and Allyson Pollock have shown, there were just 11,000 recipients of Income Support in private and third sector nursing and residential homes in 1979, at a cost of £10 million per year.[8] By February 1993, the figures had reached almost 300,000 people and a cost of £2.6 billion per year.[9]

This rise is hardly surprising. The 1980s saw a significant squeeze on local government budgets. Many local authority leaders were relieved to have the opportunity to use a central department's budget to fulfil statutory social care duties. In some cases, people were actively encouraged to use the social security system to pay for care in a private sector care home. In others, local authorities engineered bureaucratic assessments, to encourage people to seek much quicker independent sector alternatives.

The *National Health Service and Community Care Act* 1990 followed,[10] enacting Griffiths' idea of a fundamental redefinition of the role of the public sector. Funding for social care devolved from central government to local government. The transition came with a new role for local authorities – as Griffiths has postulated, they became brokers, rather than providers, of care.[11] To ensure dominance of the independent provider sector, and that local authorities did not take the opportunity to deliver better, cheaper care directly, a new Special Transition Grant was made available for personal care, with a stipulation that at least 85 per cent of the money would be spent on private sector providers.[12]

At the time, these reforms were framed as a move towards a 'mixed economy' of social care provision. In reality, it delivered near total dominance of social care provision by the independent sector. In 1979, about two thirds of residential and nursing home beds were provided by either local authorities or the NHS. In 1993, 95 per cent of domiciliary care was provided by local authorities. By 2012, the numbers were 6 and 11 per cent respectively.[13]

NEOLIBERAL CARE TODAY

The care system's neoliberalism has only increased in the subsequent decades. The market share of the private sector continues to tick up year on year. Analysis by the IPPR and Future Care Capital found a 2 per cent increase in private sector provision between 2015 and 2019 (though this might not sound like a huge increase, the increase comes from an existing position of private sector dominance).[14]

As significant as the market share of the private sector is the increasing shift in the market – from small providers, better embedded in the communities they serve, to large providers. As in many other parts of the country's economy, small, family-run providers are being pushed out by large, faceless corporations. The most recent analysis shows that five big providers control almost one fifth of the social care sector.[15] Behind them, the relative market share of companies with fleets of at least 50 care homes is growing, while small companies overseeing one or a few local residential homes are struggling.[16]

The shift to large providers has come alongside a significant shift to provision by firms funded through private equity. At the time of writing, the five biggest companies are: HC-One Limited (5.1 per cent market share); Four Seasons (3.7 per cent market share); Barchester Health-care (3.3 per cent market share); Care UK (2.4 per cent market share) and BUPA Group (2.2 per cent market share). That gives the five biggest providers control of almost 20 per cent of all for-profit social care beds. Three of these are owned by private equity (HC-One, Four Seasons and Care UK).[17] One more is a public company with ultimate shareholder registration in Jersey, a tax haven (Barchester Healthcare).

This shift from a public to a private delivery model in social care will be, for many, sufficient enough evidence to justify a major and radical reform project. But in making the popular case, it's important to go one step further – and to fully outline how the shift has translated into negative outcomes: for people, for the sector and for workers.

LOW QUALITY, LOW ACCESS, HIGH COST

The shift towards big, private equity funded care provision has come with direct implications for quality of care.[18] There is evidence that private providers offer lower levels of training and lower rates of workforce pay than their voluntary and public counterparts. In turn, they have higher rates of staff turnover and lower overall levels of staffing.[19] Other studies, including one by the sector's inspector, the Care Quality Commission, have shown that a smaller, less well-trained workforce translates to a measurable impact on the quality-of-care provision provided.[20]

It's unsurprising, then, that there is a link between the size of a provider and the quality of care it provides. 89 per cent of small nursing and residential homes have either a good or outstanding rating from the Care Quality Commission. In large residential care homes, the figure is 72 per cent good or outstanding, and in large nursing homes the figure is just 65 per cent.[21] Worse, there are hundreds of care providers that have never had a rating better than 'requires improvement'.[22] That is a remarkable differential in quality of care. It indicates the human consequences of how the social care system has evolved over the last four decades, and also demonstrates how many people could find themselves receiving inadequate levels of support if further shifts to larger, more heavily financialised big corporate providers are allowed to continue.

Poor care is the tip of the iceberg. A lack of public investment over decades in social care has meant, in essence, a system designed only to provide care for those with the very greatest need. Funds only become available when people have deteriorated – when their needs have become far more intensive – rather than when an intervention could still maintain their health and independence.[23] As many as nine in ten local authorities in England only provide care for people who have either 'substantial' or 'critical' needs.[24]

This means there are huge levels of unmet need across the country. In 2018, I released research while at Macmillan Cancer Support that quantified this for the cohort of people living with cancer. That analysis showed that as many as two in three people living with cancer had practical care needs – but that only a fraction was getting adequate levels of support. When asked about the support they needed within their homes, 38 per cent of people on a low income and 19 per cent of people on a high income had unmet needs. When asked about the support they needed outside of their homes, 34 per cent of people on a low income and 13 per cent of people on a high income had unmet needs.[25]

More broadly, a comprehensive review of unmet needs in adult social care by the Centre for Analysis of Social Exclusion found 1.5 million adults living in England and over 65 with at least one unmet care need – leaving them without the support needed to live a good life.[26] Age UK predicts this will rise to 2.1 million by 2030, without intervention.[27] And while there is no equivalent figure for people under 65, analysis by the Health Foundation shows that 35 per cent of the requests made by people aged 18 to 64 are rejected by their local authority.[28]

This underwhelming system comes with a significant cost. Under the current system, people pay until they no longer have assets worth £23,250. This means a great many people lose almost all of their wealth, over the course of their lifetime. According to the charity Independent Age, around 143,000 older people face the prospect of paying 'catastrophic lifetime costs' of £100,000 or more – around one in three people within the residential care system.[29]

It's a hugely regressive system. In essence, it is designed to take *all* the wealth of most, working people who have the poor fortune to need help when they get older – while leaving the finances of the very richest broadly intact.[30] In practice, it operates as a 100 per cent inheritance tax for those with the least money, with the proceeds going into private profits rather than the state. It is a system that keeps the poor, poor and the richest, rich – across generations.

The regressive nature of our social care system looks set to continue. In September 2021, the government announced a 'new plan' for social care. Under this plan, people will pay up to £86,000 for their social care (over their life)[31] – and they'll only pay if their total wealth is under £125,000. This is scheduled to come into effect from Autumn 2023. But this will still leave us with a system that benefits the wealthiest. Modelling of this system has shown:

- A person with a house valued at £125,000, receiving 5 years of social care, would spend 49 per cent of their wealth on care – leaving them at clear risk of financial ruin
- A person with a house valued at £500,000, receiving 5 years of social care, would spend only 17 per cent of their total wealth on social care – leaving their finances broadly intact

That is, even once this new policy comes into effect, it will still mean a social care system that operates on the brutal logic of American healthcare.

CHRONIC PROVIDER FRAGILITY

Another consequence relates to the stability of the providers who deliver services. Indeed, the current private equity-dominated social care system bears comparison to the Private Finance Initiatives (PFI) that were widely criticised when extensively used by the NHS between 1992 and 2018.[32]

The mechanics of PFI worked as follows. NHS trusts would put out a tender, asking for expressions of interest from private sector contractors, to build new health capital assets. These tenders would be for large projects – such as the construction of new hospitals. Bids would then come from consortiums, with successful parties forming a 'special purchase vehicle'. The consortium would then, usually, fund the construction of the hospital using large amounts of debt. The NHS would not face any costs until the build was complete. But once it was, they would begin paying 'unitary payments' – an annual charge that was meant to cover the risk taken by the private sector, but which in reality saw individual NHS trusts pay significantly inflated fees.[33]

The risks associated with this model of public–private partnership were epitomised in 2018 when Carillion – one of the biggest PFI beneficiaries – collapsed. It immediately left behind £7bn of debt, 3,000 lost jobs within the company and a further 75,000 impacted jobs within its supply chain.[34]

While the government have since committed to ending PFI procurement, the problem is not the scheme per se, but the relationship between the state and the private sector it represents – broadly the same relationship that defines the relationship seen in the social care market. As with PFI, here the state underwrites guaranteed payments, supporting large private sector profits. To maximise those profits, social care providers often look to expand through extensive use of debt and other high-risk business practices. The resulting system is defined by its expense to the taxpayer, a lack of quality as the sector looks to maximise profit and a lack of provider stability that often leads to high profile collapses.

Social care has been host to a number of big, 'Carillion-style' collapses. Most recently, the Four Seasons Healthcare provider went into administration, putting the care of 17,000 residents at risk, as well as the jobs of 22,000 employees. In 2011, major operator Southern Cross also collapsed after just 15 years of operation, 9 of which had seen it owned by venture capital firms.

The story of Southern Cross is illuminating. Before its collapse it had been in the middle of a significant expansion. It quickly became the largest operator in the sector. Rapid expansion led to large profits for investors and very generous salaries for the executive team. One executive sold his individual stake in the company for a substantial £36.6 million (550p a share). Just months after this transaction, Southern Cross announced its first profit warning.[35] By July 2011, it announced its closure – news that left the residents of its 752 care homes with a very real threat of homelessness hanging over them.[36.]

The closure comes down to the strategy Southern Cross used to expand as quickly as it did. It had worked on the basis of building properties, selling them off and then leasing them – a concept known as 'sell and leaseback'. As a practice, this is a high-risk, high-reward method of increasing liquidity – enabling expansion. In the end, Southern Cross could not sustain the liquid funds needed to meet its huge running costs – nor could it provide the quality of services needed to retain sufficient resident numbers. That doesn't mean their approach didn't make some people very rich in the meantime. It wasn't investors or executives who lost out. It was workers, service users and the taxpayer.

Southern Cross were not trying to go bankrupt, nor were the other care providers who have failed. Rather, their strategy was to make as much money as possible, as quickly as possible. Those running and profiting from Southern Cross didn't face any of the risk and consequences of such a high-risk strategy. It was the state and care home residents that paid the price of their strategy, designed around profit extraction rather than high quality public service.

Carillion's collapse was equally a collapse linked to a crisis of liquidity, brought about by an unsustainable reach for fast profits. The PFI construction company recycled its own liquidity, by selling its interests in hospitals to investment companies quickly after completing construction – creating funds that could be pumped into expansion and help to maximise profit extraction.

When this instability isn't causing the country's largest adult social care providers to collapse, it can be linked to alarming stories of negligence. An indicative example emerged in at the Whitchurch Care Home in January 2019. A visit from the sector's inspector exposed:

> Widespread and systemic failings . . . during the inspection. The quality and safety monitoring systems used by the provider were not fully effective. They did not ensure that there were the right resources in place to ensure the quality-of-service provision and mitigate risks to people.[37]

Systematic failings include the failure to fix an elevator, meaning second floor residents couldn't be transferred to ambulances; people regularly going without their prescribed medication; and 'occasions when people's dignity had been compromised'.[38] This was a care home being run at the very lowest possible price, under huge financial pressure, trying to remain afloat. In this case, as in so many others, the care providers failed to do so. Whitchurch care home's owner – Four Seasons Healthcare – entered administration three months later.

WORKFORCE EXPLOITATION

While researching this book, I was fortunate to have the chance to hear from social care workers directly about their experiences of working in the sector. During the second Covid lockdown, I talked to Jenny.[39] Jenny had left social care and was happy for her story to be shared.

Jenny had been drawn into social care when looking for a job where she could genuinely help people. Having enjoyed another, short period of employment in the sector – working for a charity in the South West of England – she took a role with a private operator after making a move to London. After just over a year struggling through her role, longer than many others manage, Jenny left the sector altogether.

The first thing Jenny talked me through was the low pay, a universal issue for the social care workforce:

> I was paid about £8 an hour. That's not enough to live on, certainly if you're paying London rent. It cost about £1.50 for the bus each way, and I could end up taking 2 or 3 bus trips an hour.

The base rate of pay is low, but Jenny told me she had at least known this was the case when she accepted the job. A more difficult and unexpected problem was the unpaid time between her appointments with clients: